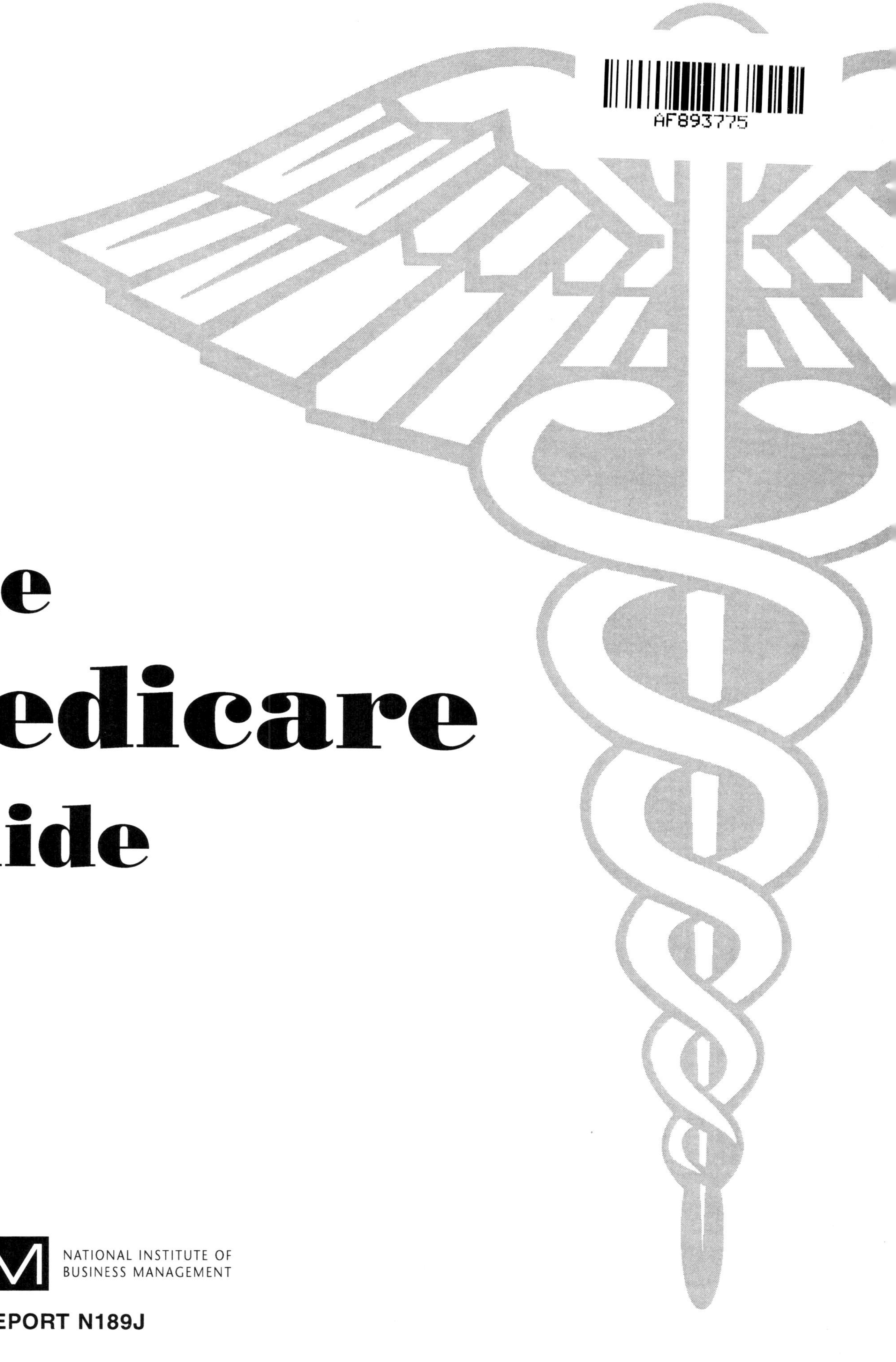

The Medicare Guide

NIBM NATIONAL INSTITUTE OF BUSINESS MANAGEMENT

SPECIAL REPORT N189J

Author
Donald J. Korn

Editor
Kathy A. Shipp

Editorial Director
Joe McGavin

Publisher
Steve Sturm

ISBN 1-880024-07-1

Contents

Medicare Reforms

As 2003 drew to a close, Congress passed the most sweeping overhaul of Medicare since the plan was created in 1965. For the first time, coverage for prescription drugs will be available to all Medicare participants. Various other changes will also have a major impact on Medicare, including a larger role for private health plans.

Under the Medicare Prescription Drug, Improvement and Modernization Act of 2003, seniors will see several changes in the next few years:

- **Discount drug cards:** Until the prescription drug benefit takes effect in 2006, Medicare participants will be able to purchase drug discount cards approved by the government, starting in spring 2004. Preliminary estimates are that the cards (sold by private companies) will cost $30 or less and save consumers up to 25 percent off the price of prescriptions.

Individuals with incomes of less than $12,124 a year or married couples with incomes below $16,363 will receive a $600 credit on their drug cards in 2004 and 2005.

- **Prescription drug benefit:** Beginning in 2006, all Medicare participants will have access to a voluntary prescription drug benefit plan. If they're in traditional Medicare, they can sign up for a separate drug benefit plan or they can join an HMO, PPO or other private plan that covers drugs as well as other medical costs.

Those in traditional Medicare may enroll in a private drug plan in which they'll pay about $35 per month in premiums, with about a $250 annual deductible. The plan will pay 75 percent of their prescription costs up to $2,250. Then there will be no coverage until a beneficiary's expenses reach $3,600. At that point the plan will pick up 95 percent of the costs, thus providing protection against catastrophic drug bills.

Estimates indicate that enrolling in a drug benefit plan will pay off for those who spend more than $800 per month on prescriptions: Their spending would drop by about 60 percent. (Low-income seniors will receive subsidies for their drug costs.)

- **Medicare Advantage:** This new, expanded program will replace Medicare+Choice *(see page 53)*. Within Medicare Advantage, private plans such as HMOs and PPOs will cover drugs as well as other medical costs.

- **Employer plans:** Some retirees now receive prescription drug coverage through their former employer's health plan. The new law provides subsidies to such employers to encourage them to maintain drug coverage for retirees.
- **More screenings:** Starting in 2005, Medicare will pay for an initial physical exam for all new Medicare beneficiaries. Also, screening for diabetes and cardiovascular disease will be covered for the first time.
- **Premiums tied to income:** Starting in 2007, upper-income Medicare beneficiaries will have to pay higher premiums for Part B coverage of doctors' visits and outpatient services.
- **Price competition:** In 2010, the government will begin a controversial six-year test of market competition. Private health plans will be allowed to compete directly with Medicare for patients based on price in six metropolitan regions.
- **Generic drugs and imports:** The new law aims to speed less expensive generic drugs to market by limiting the ability of pharmaceutical companies to create delays. However, the ban on importing less expensive drugs from Canada will remain in effect.
- **Medical Savings Accounts:** The new law makes these "medical IRAs" a permanent option for Medicare participants. MSAs are tax-advantaged accounts typically used in conjunction with catastrophic (high-deductible) health insurance. *(See Section 5.)*

* * *

Until most of these changes kick in around 2006, Medicare participants will continue to have two basic options: participate in the traditional, fee-for-service plan and buy a drug discount card or join a Medicare HMO that covers drug costs.

Fee-for-Service: Traditional but Costly

If you choose to enroll in traditional Medicare, you can pick your own doctors and hospitals. With this option, though, you may incur considerable out-of-pocket costs because traditional Medicare won't cover all your medical bills.

The average out-of-pocket costs for beneficiaries in traditional fee-for-service Medicare exceed $2,600 per year, according to the Commonwealth Fund, a private foundation supporting independent research on health and social issues. That $2,600 includes Medicare premiums, deductibles, co-payments and items not covered by Medicare currently, such as prescription drugs. However, the figure does not include the cost of long-term care provided at home or in a nursing home.

Prescription drugs alone cost Medicare beneficiaries an average of $798 out of pocket in 2003, according to the Commonwealth Fund. While Americans 65 and older represent about 13 percent of the population, they take more than one-third of all the prescription drugs sold annually in the United States. Yet Medicare does not yet pay a penny toward outpatient prescriptions. (As mentioned above, until the voluntary drug benefit kicks in, discount drug cards may save you money in 2004 and 2005.)

To protect yourself against these extraordinary costs, you may want to supplement traditional Medicare with a Medigap policy. Such policies (described in Section 4) will pick up a large share of your out-of-pocket costs, but they can be expensive. For example, in 2003, the average premium for a Medigap policy was $1,412 a year for a 65-year-old woman, according to Weiss Ratings.

HMOs: Economical but Restrictive

Until traditional Medicare includes a prescription drug benefit, seniors seeking relief may still turn to HMOs. Currently, 70 percent of those enrolled in Medicare HMOs receive some drug benefit coverage.

A Commonwealth Fund study found that seniors enrolled in Medicare HMOs in 2003 spent an average of $1,964 a year on health care. While this amount is significant, it's still about 25 percent less than the average spent by those in traditional Medicare ($2,631). In addition, many seniors in traditional Medicare also bought a Medigap policy, which on average cost $1,412, as noted above.

When you enroll in a Medicare HMO, you don't need to buy a Medigap policy because the HMO is obligated to provide comprehensive coverage. Many HMOs cover services that go beyond those provided by traditional Medicare or Medigap policies, such as dental and vision care.

The tradeoff, though, is a lack of control over your health care. When you enroll in a Medicare HMO, you basically agree to use the doctors, hospitals and

Medicare's Future Health

In its 2003 annual report, the Medicare Board of Trustees projected that the program would run out of money by 2026, four years earlier than it estimated in 2002. This speedup in the expected day of reckoning was blamed on projections of lower revenues and higher expenditures.

As recently as 1998, however, the trustees had predicted that Medicare would run out of money by 2008. Thus, the picture is still brighter than it was six years ago.

In the 2003 report, the projected year when Medicare expenditures would exceed tax revenues was pushed forward three years, from 2015 to 2012, but that's still two years later than estimated in the 2000 report. Thus, the short- and medium-term outlook for Medicare remains encouraging.

Over the long run, though, Medicare's hospital insurance trust fund fails by a wide margin to meet the test of financial balance. Future outlays are projected to outstrip revenues. As a result, the trustees' report calls for further reform: "The financial difficulties facing Social Security and Medicare are not insurmountable, but we must take action to address them in a timely manner. The sooner they are addressed, the more varied and less disruptive can be their solutions."

However, the 2003 Medicare law adds still more financial obligations to a program that faces serious long-term difficulties.

other providers inside the network. You may not be permitted to see a specialist unless your primary care physician gives you a referral. Moreover, many Medicare HMOs are cutting back on the services they offer, raising their charges or dropping out of Medicare altogether. As a result, enrollees have found themselves in a position of paying more for fewer benefits. Some beneficiaries have been forced to change Medicare HMOs, disrupting their lives; others have had to return to traditional Medicare because no HMO was available in their area.

The information provided in this Special Report can help you decide whether the benefits of Medicare HMOs are worth the restrictions and the risks of further cutbacks and dropouts. Although the new Medicare law raises the reimbursement rates for Medicare HMOs, it remains to be seen whether more money will encourage more HMOs to enter the program.

Although Medicare HMOs have lost ground since their popularity peaked in the late 1990s, they continue to retain their enrollment figures. In 2004, about 11 percent of Medicare enrollees are in HMOs, compared to 5 percent in 1993.

Its Historical Perspective

When Medicare was enacted in 1965, the federal health insurance program covered most people age 65 and older. In 1972 coverage was extended to include certain disabled individuals and those suffering from permanent kidney failure. Another change at that time made it possible for individuals who otherwise would not be covered by Medicare to elect to buy into the program. Currently, Medicare serves more than 40 million older and disabled Americans. Many of those covered by Medicare have annual incomes of $25,000 or less. Each year, Medicare handles about 800 million claims for roughly one million hospitals, doctors and medical equipment suppliers.

Medicare's huge, complex system is administered by the Centers for Medicare & Medicaid Services (CMS), an agency of the U.S. Department of Health and Human Services. CMS sets the standards that hospitals, skilled nursing facilities, home health agencies, hospices and other providers and suppliers of health care services must meet in order to receive payment for Medicare-covered services. The Social Security Administration (SSA) provides beneficiary services: enrollment applications, inquiries and collection of premiums.

The Medicare program has two parts, hospital insurance coverage (Part A) and medical insurance coverage (Part B), as defined in Title XVIII of the Social Security Act of 1965. Basically, Part A pays for health care provided in hospitals, skilled nursing facilities and hospices, as well as some skilled nursing care in your home. Part B pays for doctors' bills, outpatient services, durable medical equipment and a number of other medical services and supplies that Part A doesn't cover.

Keep in mind that Medicare was never intended to be a comprehensive health insurance program. You'll need to assess your personal situation so you can assemble a total health insurance package tailored to your needs.

1

Medicare Basics

Medicare is a voluntary program, open to any U.S. citizen or legal permanent resident age 65 or older. Additionally, certain younger individuals who meet the requirements of Social Security's disability program or have permanent kidney failure are eligible for benefits. You cannot be barred from Medicare on account of pre-existing health conditions, nor can you be charged more for Medicare because of your age or health status.

In 2003 Medicare paid about $268 billion in benefits. Payments in 2004 are projected to be roughly $284 billion. Even if you are not currently on Medicare, as a taxpayer you are affected by this vast program. The financing for Part A (hospital insurance) comes primarily from payroll taxes. Only about 25 percent of the financing for Part B (supplementary medical insurance) comes from the monthly premiums of those who enroll in the program; the remainder comes from the general revenues of the federal government. Thus the government's tax and spending policies have implications for everyone.

How Payroll Taxes Work

Although Social Security and Medicare are technically separate taxes (Social Security covers retirement, survivors' and disability benefits), for the most part they are simply added together and treated as one payroll tax.

Every employer must withhold from the employee's pay not only federal income tax but also the combined Social Security and Medicare tax and then make these payments to the government (or a designated bank). IRS Form 941 is used to report the federal taxes withheld and the employer's matching portion of the combined Social Security and Medicare tax. Small business owners usually have to make these payments at least quarterly. So whether you are an employer or an employee, you pay taxes for Social Security and Medicare, and the taxes come right out of your income. Self-employed persons pay these taxes through their quarterly estimated or annual income tax payments.

In 2004, the combined employee-employer tax rate for Social Security and Medicare is the same as it was in 2003: 7.65 percent (6.2 percent for Social Security and 1.45 percent for Medicare). Currently, you do not pay any tax for Social Security on any earnings over the maximum taxable amount, which in 2004 is $87,900, compared with $87,000 in 2003. There is, however, no cap on earnings for the Medicare portion of the tax. For self-employed individuals, the tax is 15.3 percent (12.4 percent for Social Security and 2.9 percent for Medicare); however, that 15.3 percent tax is assessed on 92.35 percent of their net annual income, up to the maximum earnings limit.

All wages and salaries (including bonuses and commissions) are taxed and credited to your earnings record. It is important that your earnings record with the Social Security Administration be accurate because your future Social Security benefits and eligibility for premium-free Medicare Part A hospital insurance will be based on this record. Starting in 1999, the SSA began mailing an earnings and benefit estimate statement to all workers age 25 and older who are not already receiving Social Security benefits. You can expect to receive your Social Security Statement every year about three months prior to your birthday. If you do not receive your statement, call the SSA at (800) 772-1213.

The Nanny Tax Law

Annual wages of $1,400 or more that you pay during 2004 to household workers age 18 and older, including nannies and baby sitters, are subject to Social Security and Medicare payroll taxes. You are required to report and pay your share of the payroll taxes, along with the taxes you withheld from your employee's wages, when you file your federal income tax return (Form 1040). *Exception:* Working students under age 18 are exempt from the tax, as are other household employees under age 18 if they have another principal occupation.

There are several deadlines you must meet to avoid possible penalties in addition to overdue taxes:

- Make sure to give your household worker copies of B, C and 2 of IRS Form W-2 (Wage and Tax Statement) by **Jan. 31** after the year in which you paid the wages.
- Send copy A of your household worker's IRS Form W-2 to the Social Security Administration by the **last day of February**.
- Pay the payroll taxes when you file your federal income tax return (Form 1040) by **April 15**.

For more information about coverage of household workers, call Social Security at (800) 772-1213 and ask for the "Household Workers" fact sheet (Publication 05-10021) or visit ***www.ssa.gov***. Or you can call the IRS at (800) 829-3676 and ask for IRS Publication 926 ("Employment Taxes for Household Employers"). Detailed instructions for completing the Form W-2 are available in IRS Notice 587 ("Preparing Form W-2 for Your Household Employee") online at ***www.irs.gov***.

To acquire credit for benefits, a person needs a certain number of "quarters of coverage" (QCs). The total earnings in a calendar year determine quarters of coverage. The amount of wages needed in 2004 to earn one quarter of coverage, or Social Security "credit," is $900. Thus, if you earn at least $3,600 ($900 multiplied by 4) in 2004, you will acquire four QCs, the maximum number that can be credited per year. (In 2002 the QC amount was $870, and in 2003, $890.)

For years before 1978, QCs were determined by a different method. For your earnings before 1978, you are entitled to one credit for each quarter in which you were paid $50 or more in wages, or four quarters of coverage for every taxable year in which you earned $400 or more of self-employment income. In general, a worker's wages are covered beginning with the first dollar paid. Beginning in 1978, the law provided that a QC would be credited for each $250 of a person's total wages and self-employment income, up to a maximum of four QCs per year. The QC amount is raised each year to keep up with average wage increases. Once you have accumulated credit for 10 years' work (40 QCs), you are "fully insured" for retirement and survivors' benefits and Medicare Part A, even if you never work again.

Besides the major revamping of Medicare in 2006, keep in mind that many minor changes are made to Medicare laws and regulations virtually every year. If you're covered by Medicare, you'll want to keep track of the amounts of premiums and deductibles, as well as covered and noncovered services, to ensure that any supplemental insurance you purchase blends well with Medicare coverage. As new Medicare benefits are introduced or others possibly eliminated, insurers will modify their plans and premiums. Each year, you should evaluate these changes and decide whether to renew, purchase, upgrade or drop policies, according to the state of your health and your financial situation.

Medicare Eligibility

Who can get Part A (hospital insurance)

People who are age 65 or older. Generally, if you or your spouse (including a divorced or deceased spouse) worked long enough to be eligible for benefits from Social Security or the Railroad Retirement Board, you are eligible for premium-free Medicare Part A (hospital insurance). Except under certain conditions, your spouse must be at least 62 years old but does not have to apply for benefits in order for you to be eligible based on his work record. In addition, a dependent parent may be eligible for Medicare Part A, based on your work record, when he turns 65.

People who are under age 65. You are eligible for Part A if you have been receiving Social Security disability payments for at least 24 months or have worked long enough in a federal, state or local government job and meet the requirements of the Social Security disability program. If you receive a disability annuity from the Railroad Retirement Board, you will be eligible for Part A after a waiting period. Disabled widows and widowers (including certain divorced widows and widowers) and disabled children may be eligible for Part A, usually after a 24-month qualifying period.

Note: For disabled widows or widowers, previous months of eligibility for Supplemental Security Income (SSI) based on disability may count toward the qualifying period.

Those with permanent kidney failure. You are eligible for Medicare Part A at any age if you are a kidney transplant or dialysis patient, and (1) you are insured or are getting monthly benefits under Social Security or the Railroad Retirement system, or (2) you have worked long enough in the federal, state or local government to be insured for Medicare. In addition, your spouse or child may be eligible, based on your work record, if she receives maintenance dialysis or has had a kidney transplant, even if no one else in the family is getting Medicare. For further information, you can obtain a copy of "Medicare Coverage of Kidney Dialysis and Kidney Transplant Services" (Publication 587-X) from any Social Security office or by writing to Medicare Publications, Centers for Medicare & Medicaid Services, 7500 Security Boulevard, Baltimore, MD 21244-1850, or to the Consumer Information Center, Department WWW, Pueblo, CO 81009.

Certain older or disabled people who do not qualify for Part A under the rules described above may be able to get coverage by paying a monthly premium *(see page 10)*. To find out whether you are eligible, call or visit your nearest Social Security office. If you are told you are ineligible, yet you believe otherwise, don't give up. Send a certified, return-receipt letter to your Social Security office asking for a written statement explaining your ineligibility. If you still disagree, contact your legal or financial adviser or your congressional representative.

Who can get Part B (medical insurance)

Almost anyone who is age 65 or older—or under age 65 but eligible for Medicare Part A—can enroll for Part B by paying a monthly premium. You don't need any Social Security or government work credits to qualify for this portion of Medicare.

Aliens who are age 65 or older and are not eligible for Part A must be legal permanent residents who have lived here for five years before they can enroll for Medicare Part B.

Enrollment: Don't Delay Sign-Up

Enrollment in Medicare is voluntary, but there is an initial enrollment period during which you should sign up to avoid a delay in obtaining coverage or incurring a possible penalty. The initial enrollment period is seven months, which begins three months before your 65th birthday, includes the month you turn 65 and ends three months after that birthday.

Note: Although we think of ourselves as turning "a year older" on our birthday, the government treats us as having attained a certain age on the day preceding our birthday. Thus a person whose 65th birthday falls on the first of the month attains 65 on the last day of the preceding month. For example, Jay Smith's

Your Medicare Card

Your Medicare card shows your coverage for Part A hospital insurance and Part B medical insurance and the date when your protection started. It also shows your health insurance claim number, which is sometimes referred to as your Medicare number.

The claim number usually has nine digits and one or two letters, sometimes followed by another number. You must always include your full claim number on all Medicare claims and correspondence. When a husband and wife both have Medicare, each receives a separate card and claim number. Each spouse must use the exact name and claim number shown on the card.

It also is important that you remember to:

- Use your Medicare card only after the effective date shown on it.
- Be sure to carry it with you when you are away from home.
- Always show your Medicare card when you get health care services.
- Always write your complete health insurance claim number (including any letters) on all checks for Medicare premium payments or any correspondence.
- Have your Medicare card available when you make a telephone inquiry.
- Immediately ask Social Security for a new card if yours is lost. You can request a replacement card online at ***www.ssa.gov*** or by calling (800) 772-1213.
- Never let anyone else use your card.

65th birthday is July 1, but he will attain age 65 in June. Therefore, his initial enrollment period for Medicare will be March 1 through Sept. 30.

If you're receiving Social Security retirement or disability benefits or Railroad Retirement checks, the SSA will automatically send you a Medicare card. Usually, the card will show that you are entitled to both Part A and Part B and will indicate the beginning dates of each. (If you are entitled to Part A insurance but are living in Puerto Rico or elsewhere outside the United States, you will not be automatically enrolled in Part B. In that case, you must file a written request.)

If you do not want Part B, for which you must pay a monthly premium, you can refuse it by following the instructions that come with the card. You also may decide to withdraw from Part B at a later date. If you voluntarily terminate your enrollment in Part B after your coverage has started, your coverage (and premium liability) will continue until the last day of the month following the month in which you filed the termination request.

If you are at least 65 and eligible for Social Security retirement benefits but don't plan to retire, you can sign up for Medicare Parts A and B without applying for monthly benefits. (A person enrolled in Part A who is age 65 or older, working and covered by an employer's health plan can postpone enrollment in Part B without penalty. You will have a special enrollment period of seven months after you retire.)

➤ **Recommendation:** If you are not already getting Social Security retirement or disability benefits or Railroad Retirement checks, be sure to contact the SSA about three months before you turn 65 to sign up for Medicare. Delaying enrollment will postpone the start of your Part A coverage by one to three months. If you don't sign up for Part B coverage during that initial period, there could be more than a year's delay in the start of your coverage. In addition, your monthly premium will increase 10 percent for each 12-month period you were eligible but did not enroll. Medicare applications and enrollment forms are available at all Social Security offices. You can file the application in person or by phone.

You should also contact Social Security about applying for Medicare in the following situations:

- **You are a disabled widow or widower** between ages 50 and 65 but have not applied for disability benefits because you already are getting another kind of Social Security benefit.
- **You are a federal, state or local government employee** and became disabled before age 65.
- **You, your spouse or your dependent child** has permanent kidney failure.
- **You turned down Medicare Part B** insurance when you became entitled to Medicare Part A.

If You Have to Buy Part A

If you are 65 or older and don't qualify for Medicare, you can buy Part A coverage, much like private insurance, by paying a monthly premium. In 2004 the monthly Part A premium for uninsured individuals age 65 and over is $343, a $27 increase from the amount in 2003. The same premium applies to certain disabled people who have exhausted other benefits (that is, their benefits ended solely because they had earnings exceeding the allowable amount for substantial gainful activity).

As we noted earlier, to qualify for Medicare, a person needs 40 quarters of coverage (QCs). If you have fewer than 30 QCs, you will have to pay the monthly premium of $343 for Medicare Part A in 2004. For those who have between 30 and 39 QCs, the monthly premium is 45 percent less, or $189 per month. The Part B premium for Medicare medical insurance in 2004 is $66.60 per month for *all* enrollees.

You may be eligible for the reduced (45 percent discount) monthly premium of $189 if you meet one of the following conditions:

- You have earned between 30 and 39 quarters of coverage based on your own work record.
- You had been married for the previous one-year period to an individual who had earned at least 30 quarters of coverage.
- You had been married for at least one year at the time of your spouse's death, and your spouse had earned at least 30 quarters of coverage.

- You are divorced from an individual who at the time of divorce had earned at least 30 quarters of coverage, and the marriage lasted at least 10 years.

If you want to buy Part A hospital insurance, you must enroll in Part B and pay a monthly premium for that coverage, too. (In this case, you can cancel Part A and still continue to buy Part B.)

If you wait to buy Part A until after the initial seven-month enrollment period, you can sign up during the general enrollment period, which is Jan. 1 through March 31. The 10 percent surcharge for late enrollment described earlier for Part B also applies to buying Part A.

However, if you have been covered under an HMO, you can buy Part A hospital insurance at any time while you are in the HMO and up to eight months after the HMO coverage has ended. The premium surcharge, if any, may be waived because of your coverage under the HMO.

If You Delayed Enrolling in Part B

Q. I didn't need Medicare's medical insurance when I turned 65, but now I do. How do I enroll?

A. If you have Part A Medicare hospital insurance but not Part B medical insurance, you can sign up for the latter during the general enrollment period (Jan. 1 through March 31 each year). Your protection will begin July 1 of the year you enroll.

Note: Unless you delayed enrolling because you were covered by an employer health plan (at the time you first became eligible for Medicare), you will be penalized for having waited to sign up. Your premium will be increased by 10 percent for each 12-month period that you delayed enrollment.

Example: Say you could have enrolled in Part B in February 2003, but you waited until February 2004. Instead of paying the 2004 monthly premium of $66.60, you would pay $73.30 a month.

Exception: If you've been covered by an employer plan and then stop working, you do not have to wait for the general enrollment period and you will not be penalized for late enrollment. You can sign up for Part B any time during a special eight-month period that begins with the month you no longer are covered by your former employer, or with the month that the employment on which the health plan is based ends, whichever is earlier.

In the case of certain disability beneficiaries, the special period begins when Medicare replaces the employer group health plan as the primary payer of those individuals' covered medical expenses.

Special enrollment period rules do not apply to you if you stop working or lose group health plan coverage during the initial enrollment period (the seven months starting three months before your 65th birthday).

➤ **Recommendation:** Contact Social Security as soon as your employment ends, or the plan coverage ends or changes, to obtain information about enrolling in Part B.

Example: You retired as a federal worker at age 65 and have an HMO under your retiree plan. After spending a full year fishing, you've gone to work for a private company. You choose to hold onto your federal retiree plan (HMO coverage) and elect to take the very minimum health plan with your private employer to complement your HMO coverage. When you retire from your current job, you will get hit with the 10 percent penalty if you enroll in Part B because you could have enrolled during the year you spent fishing. However, signing up for your health plan at work should stop the clock from increasing any penalty you might face later. Furthermore, if you keep your federal HMO indefinitely, you might decide not to sign up for Part B at all, which is always your option.

Note: Although you were covered by an HMO when you first were able to get Medicare, you will be hit with the premium surcharge if you decide to drop the HMO coverage and enroll in Part A because the HMO coverage was not based on current employment.

Keep a Paper Trail

- **Your Medicare card** is essential to obtaining your benefits. Always carry your card with you, and always show it when you receive covered services.
- **Fill out the form** on page 13 (or create a similar form), and keep it in an accessible place. Include all your Medicare and health insurance information to make it easy for you—or someone else in the event of an illness or accident—to locate important data quickly. Store your policy in a safe place, and keep it up to date.
- **If you have to apply for Medicare,** be sure to do so during the initial enrollment period, which begins three months before you turn 65.
- **As inconvenient as it may be,** keep a detailed "paper trail." Write your health insurance number on any correspondence related to Medicare. Send all correspondence by certified mail, return receipt.
- **When you call your local Social Security office,** a Medicare intermediary or Medicare carrier, keep a log of all telephone calls. Note the number called, the date and time of the call, the name(s) of those who have provided you with information and a summary of the information given.
- **Keep a record** of each and every health care service you receive and all charges for such services, along with the name of the health care provider and the date you received medical care. It is a good idea to keep a chronological notebook detailing all Medicare information received and services provided.

For more information, visit Medicare's Web site at ***www.medicare.gov***.

For Your Records

Your Medicare claim number (also called your Medicare number from your card)	______
Date protection started (from your card)	______
Local Social Security office	______
Address	______
Phone	______
Contact	______
State insurance office	______
Address	______
Phone	______
Contact	______
Medicare carrier	______
Address	______
Phone	______
Contact	______
Private policy carrier	______
Address	______
Phone	______
Policy number	______
Agent's name	______
Agent's phone	______
—or—	
HMO	______
Address	______
Phone	______
Patient or account number	______

A Note About Medicaid

Many people think that Medicaid and Medicare are different names for the same program. In fact, they are different programs, although both are administered by the Department of Health and Human Services.

Medicaid is a state-run program designed primarily to help those with low incomes and little or no financial resources. Most states also cover the needy elderly, blind and disabled who receive assistance under the Supplemental Security Income (SSI) program. Coverage also is available for certain infants and low-income individuals who qualify as medically needy.

The federal government helps pay for Medicaid, but each state has its own rules about eligibility and coverage. Some people qualify for both Medicare and Medicaid. For more information about the Medicaid program, contact your local social services or welfare office or call CMS at (410) 786-3000.

Help for Low-Income Medicare Beneficiaries

If your income and assets are very limited, you may qualify for the Qualified Medicare Beneficiary (QMB) program or the Specified Low-Income Medicare Beneficiary (SLMB) program. Both are run by CMS and each state agency that provides medical assistance under Medicaid.

The programs differ in the amount of income that qualifies you for assistance. In general, you must be entitled to Medicare Part A to be eligible for either the QMB or SLMB program. If you qualify for the QMB program, your state will pay your monthly Medicare premiums. You will also not have to pay the Medicare deductibles and co-insurance. If you qualify for the SLMB program, your state will pay only for your Part B monthly premium.

The rules vary from state to state, but, in general, you may qualify for help from the QMB or SLMB program if your income (including Social Security benefits, pensions and wages) is limited and your financial resources (such as bank accounts, stocks and bonds), excluding your home, do not exceed certain limits.

Only your state can decide if you qualify for either program. Contact your state or local medical assistance (Medicaid) agency, social services office or welfare office, or call the Medicare hotline at (800) 633-4227. For general information, ask the Social Security Administration for a free copy of "Help for Low-Income Medicare Beneficiaries" (Publication 05-10079).

2

Medicare Coverage

As one might expect, the Medicare program is complicated. Medicare patients may be treated by any licensed physician. However, other suppliers—such as hospitals, HMOs, home health care services, hospices and skilled nursing facilities—must be Medicare certified to be paid by Medicare. This certification means that these health care providers must be willing to comply with a great deal of red tape, so many factors limit your choices.

For example, Part A (hospital insurance) covers treatment in hospitals and "skilled nursing" facilities, plus some of the cost for care in your home or in a hospice. However, most nursing homes are not considered skilled nursing facilities, and not all services provided by skilled nursing facilities are covered by Medicare. As a result, finding a skilled nursing facility that qualifies for reimbursement may be difficult. For Medicare purposes, it is the federal government that defines "skilled nursing" care, not you or your doctor. Moreover, the federal definitions dictate the status of the facility as well.

Who Administers Medicare

The Department of Health and Human Services has overall responsibility for administering the Medicare program, along with its various agencies, including CMS and the SSA. CMS has primary responsibility for Medicare, including policy formulation, contract oversight and operation, maintenance and review of utilization records and general financing of Medicare. The SSA is responsible for the initial determination of an individual's eligibility and maintains the master Medicare beneficiary record.

The Department of Treasury manages both the Medicare Part A and Part B trust funds and the transfer of funds to pay the bills. A board of trustees gives Congress an annual report on the status and operation of the Medicare trust funds.

Medicare payments are processed by private insurance companies that have contracts with the federal government. Companies that handle hospitalization claims (Part A) are called Medicare (or fiscal) **intermediaries**; those that handle claims for services by doctors and other suppliers (Part B) are called Medicare **carriers**. The amounts that Medicare will pay on claims are determined by detailed fee schedules, which vary across the country.

CMS enters into agreements with state agencies and the fiscal intermediaries (often Blue Cross/Blue Shield associations) to help administer the hospital insurance plan. The state agencies survey institutions to determine whether they meet the conditions for participation as a hospital, skilled nursing facility, home health agency or hospice, and they assist institutions in meeting the conditions for participation. The fiscal intermediaries determine the amount of benefits payable to the hospitals, skilled nursing facilities, hospices and home health agencies and pay benefits to those institutions out of funds advanced by the federal government. The intermediaries also assist the institutions with recordkeeping, conduct audits to ensure payments are proper, and serve as a channel of information on hospital insurance protection.

Peer review organizations (PROs) are groups of practicing doctors and other health care professionals paid by the federal government to monitor the care given to Medicare patients. Each state has a PRO, which has the authority to decide whether care given to Medicare patients is reasonable, necessary, provided in the most appropriate setting and meets standards of quality generally accepted by the medical profession. All PRO decisions are in writing and will indicate if you are responsible for payment when Medicare will not pay for a service.

Note: Medicare does not usually pay for services that are not "reasonable and necessary" for diagnosing or treating an illness or injury. Services for which Medicare may not pay include the following:

- Drugs or devices that have not been approved by the Food and Drug Administration or medical procedures and services performed using such drugs or devices.
- Services, including drugs or devices, not considered safe and effective because they are experimental. Historically, CMS has equated the term "experimental" with "investigational." However, Medicare coverage may be available for certain FDA-approved investigational devices.

Under contracts with CMS, the Medicare carriers help administer Part B, the medical insurance plan. The carriers determine the amount of insurance benefits to be paid; pay benefits from funds advanced by the federal government; ensure that the payments being made are proper; serve as a channel of information relating to the medical insurance plan; and grant a fair hearing to individuals according to established procedures. There are also special carriers called **durable medical equipment regional carriers** (DMERCs), which handle claims for durable medical equipment, oxygen and some other supplies.

Part A: Hospital Insurance

While you are a patient in a hospital, you will be covered for most basic benefits after you pay an initial deductible per benefit period. The deductible is set at $876 for 2004. In addition to inpatient hospital coverage, Part A will pay for some skilled nursing facility care, certain home health services and hospice care. (Medicare does not pay for "custodial care," such as help with dressing, walking and bathing. It is important to understand the difference between skilled nursing care and custodial care. If you are in doubt about coverage, obtain an opinion in advance, if possible, and preferably in writing.)

Q. Are there prerequisites for hospitalization coverage?

A. Provided that your treatment meets four conditions, Medicare will pay according to the schedule outlined in "Medicare Coverage at a Glance" *(see page 34)*. The four conditions are:

- A doctor must prescribe hospitalization.
- Your condition must require the kind of care that can be provided only in a hospital.
- The hospital must be a participant in Medicare.
- The Utilization Review Committee of the hospital, the local PRO or the intermediary responsible for processing the Medicare claim does not disapprove of your stay.

Q. Does Medicare cover care provided in a nursing home?

A. As noted previously, a skilled nursing facility is defined by Medicare regulations, and few nursing homes qualify for such coverage. Even then, Medicare coverage is limited in this category. The following conditions must be met:

1. **Your condition requires daily skilled nursing** or skilled rehabilitative services that, as a practical matter, can be provided only in the skilled nursing facility.
2. **You have been in a hospital at least three days** in a row (not counting the day of discharge) before being admitted to a participating skilled nursing facility.
3. **Your care in the skilled nursing facility** is for a condition that was treated in the hospital.
4. **A medical professional certifies** that you need skilled nursing or rehabilitative services daily.
5. **You are admitted to the skilled nursing facility** within a short time (usually 30 days) after leaving the hospital. The usual period may be extended when a covered level of skilled facility care would not be medically appropriate within 30 days of discharge from the hospital, and covered care will probably be needed later.

Once you've met these conditions, Medicare helps pay for 100 days per benefit period, provided that the Medicare intermediary or the skilled nursing facility's Utilization Review Committee does not disapprove of your stay.

Note: In some cases, the need for services in a skilled nursing facility may become apparent only after you have unsuccessfully tried convalescent care in your home. Similarly, if you are discharged from a skilled nursing facility, benefits may be resumed if you are readmitted (to the same or another participating skilled nursing facility) within 30 days of the discharge. But what if more than 30 days have elapsed? Benefits may not be resumed even if you have used fewer than 100 days of skilled nursing facility services in that benefit period unless (1) the later admission was medically predictable at the time of the hospital discharge or (2) you've had another qualifying hospital stay and again meet all the conditions for extended-care benefits.

Q. How is a "benefit period" defined?

A. Do not assume that a benefit period coincides with the calendar year. Benefit periods are defined in a way that lets CMS measure your use of health care services. Your first benefit period starts the first time you enter a hospital after your Medicare insurance begins. It ends when you have been out of a hospital, skilled nursing facility or rehabilitation center for at least 60 consecutive days, including the day you are discharged. It also ends if you remain in a skilled nursing facility but do not receive any skilled care there for 60 days in a row. With the exception of hospice care (discussed later in this section), there is no limit to the number of benefit periods you may have.

Q. Does Medicare pay for skilled health care at home?

A. If you require skilled health care in your home, Medicare may pay the full approved cost for an unlimited number of home care visits by a visiting nurse, physical therapist or other approved health care worker. The care you need must include "intermittent" skilled nursing care, physical therapy or other approved services (such as speech therapy and services provided by occupational therapists, home health aides and medical social workers). Prior hospitalization is not required, but you must be confined to your home and a physician must set up your home health care plan.

You will be responsible for paying for any full-time nursing costs, drugs, meals delivered to your home and homemaker services. Medicare will pay 80 percent of the approved amount for durable medical equipment, such as wheelchairs, walkers and bedside trays, provided they are prescribed by a physician.

Note: The term "intermittent care" is not the same as "hourly care," although both may be described as part time. In determining whether they are covered, Medicare looks at how often the visits occur and how long they last. Typically, intermittent visits occur as often as medically necessary, usually two to three times per week for less than an hour, but occasionally they may be daily and (although rare) even twice a day. Finally, the visits are continued only until the goals of your treatment plan are met. Usually, you must pay for hourly services yourself. Typically, visits that occur as often as you want, last as long as you want (usually there is a two-hour minimum), and continue for as long a period as you want are considered hourly services.

Under a new policy, a home health agency must send you a notice explaining why and when it expects Medicare to stop paying for your home health care. If you think Medicare should continue to pay, you can request that the home health agency send your claim to Medicare for a decision. If Medicare decides not to pay, you will receive a letter explaining how you can appeal its decision.

Q. How does custodial care differ from skilled home care?

A. Because there has been much confusion in this area, be aware that Medicare will not pay for custodial care (assistance with eating, dressing and bathing), regardless of whether it is in your home or in a skilled nursing facility. Although certain health care at home is allowed under Medicare, CMS is cracking down on unnecessary services.

Generally, if you need part-time skilled health care at home, Medicare hospital insurance will pay the full approved cost of services furnished by a participating home health agency, such as one specializing in skilled nursing and therapeutic services in the home. To qualify, five conditions must be met:

- The care you need involves intermittent skilled nursing care or physical or speech therapy.
- You are confined to your home.
- A doctor has determined that you require this care and has set up a home health plan for you.
- The home health agency participates in Medicare.
- The physician does not have a significant financial or contractual relationship with the home health agency.

Coverage for Transplants

Since 1995 Medicare has covered lung transplants performed in hospitals that have documented experience and success in performing the procedure. Under this policy, a hospital applying for approval as a Medicare Lung Transplant Center must document certain one-year and two-year survival rates for lung transplant patients.

Medicare also covers kidney, heart and liver transplants. However, the program helps pay for heart and liver transplants only when performed in facilities meeting special quality standards, such as those for lung transplants. Combined heart/lung transplants will be covered by Medicare when done in a hospital approved for either heart or lung transplants.

Other than this limited skilled home care, Medicare does not cover general household services, meal preparation, shopping or other home-care-related services. Nor does it pay for full-time nursing at home, prescription drugs (until 2006) or blood transfusions. It will pay for physical therapy and speech therapy in the home, as well as for certain occupational therapy, part-time home health aides, medical supplies, social services and 80 percent of the approved cost of physician-prescribed durable medical equipment for home use.

Because Medicare won't help pay for custodial care, that means a large gap is likely to exist in your health care coverage. Most people enter nursing homes to receive custodial care—often for chronic ailments or disabilities from which they will not recover. Long-term-care costs for custodial care may be picked up by Medicaid, but this program is available only after a patient's savings have been exhausted. *(For another alternative, see Long-Term-Care Policies in Section 6.)*

Q. Does Medicare cover hospice care?

A. In 1983 hospice care was added as a covered service for terminally ill patients with a life expectancy of six months or less. Hospice care does not focus on curative treatment; rather, it is designed to provide counseling, supportive services and pain control in a program that coordinates inpatient, outpatient and home care.

With the exception of small co-payments for outpatient drugs and inpatient respite care, Medicare provides coverage for the full cost of hospice care for those terminally ill patients who elect it *(see page 21)*. Covered services include nursing and doctors' services, drugs for pain relief and symptom management, physical therapy, home health aides, medical social services, counseling, short-

Medicare Coverage in Foreign Hospitals

Certain important exceptions to the rule barring Medicare coverage in foreign hospitals involve Mexican and Canadian hospitals. According to CMS' *Medicare Handbook*, Medicare can help pay for care in these two border countries in these situations:

- You are in the United States when an emergency occurs, and a Canadian or Mexican hospital is closer than the nearest U.S. hospital that can provide the emergency services you need.
- You live in the United States, but a Canadian or Mexican hospital that can provide the care you need is closer to your home than the nearest U.S. hospital. The situation need not be an emergency.
- You are traveling through Canada—"without unreasonable delay and by the most direct route between Alaska and another state"—when an emergency occurs, and a Canadian hospital is closer than the nearest U.S. hospital.

Medicare also pays for doctor and ambulance services in Canada or Mexico in connection with a covered inpatient hospital stay.

term inpatient care (including respite care) and homemaker services. To qualify for coverage:

- A doctor must certify that you are terminally ill.
- The care must be provided by a Medicare-certified hospice program.
- You must have selected hospice care instead of standard Medicare benefits for the terminal illness. In doing so, you have given up Medicare coverage for treatment of the illness itself. If, however, while receiving hospice care, you require treatment for a condition not related to the terminal illness, Medicare will help pay for that treatment.
- Special benefit periods apply. Medicare will pay for two 90-day periods of hospice care, followed by an unlimited number of 60-day periods, provided each period is recertified by a doctor.

As a hospice patient, you always have the right to stop getting hospice care, for whatever reason. If you stop your hospice care, you will get your health care from traditional Medicare or your Medicare HMO. If you are eligible, you can go back to hospice care at any time.

Example: Warren Dodge is a cancer patient who received hospice care for two 90-day periods before his cancer went into remission. At the start of the next 60-day period of care, his doctor decided that Warren would not need to return to hospice care at that time. If Warren becomes eligible once more, he may be recertified and can elect to return to hospice care.

There are no deductibles for hospice care. The patient is responsible for no more than $5 for each prescription drug and other similar products for pain relief and symptom control. Periodic inpatient respite care—to give relief to the person caring for the patient at home—is covered for up to five days at a time in a Medicare-approved hospital or nursing home. The patient pays 5 percent of the cost, or about $5 a day, for respite care. There is no limit to the number of times you can receive respite care, but the amount you pay for this type of care can change each year.

Q. Does Medicare cover other kinds of hospitals and sanitariums?

A. Part A of Medicare provides a lifetime coverage allotment for care in psychiatric hospitals. For 2004 that allotment is a lifetime total of 190 days of inpatient psychiatric care. Once you have used the 190 days, Part A does not pay for any more inpatient care in a psychiatric hospital. In most cases, psychiatric care in general hospitals, rather than free-standing psychiatric hospitals, is not subject to this 190-day limit. Inpatient psychiatric care in a general hospital is treated the same as other Medicare inpatient care.

There are additional limitations on the number of hospital days that Medicare will pay for, however, if you were already hospitalized for psychiatric care when you first became covered by Medicare. Contact Social Security or your Medicare intermediary for more information.

Restrictions on Cataract Surgery

Cataract surgery is the most commonly performed surgical procedure covered by the Medicare program. Analyses performed for CMS, however, have found that a number of cataract surgeries are not medically necessary.

As a result, the mere presence of a cataract does not mean that surgery is needed. If you are able to function normally or the condition can be corrected with eyeglasses, surgery may not be considered medically necessary and thus may not be covered by Medicare.

Keep in mind that not all hospitals participate in the Medicare program. Medicare may pay all or only part of certain emergency treatment in a nonparticipating hospital, and even then only if it is the nearest hospital when you became ill or had an accident.

Note: The Balanced Budget Act of 1997 authorized Medicare and Medicaid payments for services received in religious nonmedical health care institutions, such as Christian Science sanitariums, under certain conditions, specified in Section 4454 of the statute.

Q. Does Medicare cover services outside the United States?

A. Medicare generally does not pay for hospitalization or medical services rendered outside the United States. (Puerto Rico, the U.S. Virgin Islands, Guam, American Samoa and the Northern Mariana Islands are, however, included.) Under limited circumstances, services furnished in the Caribbean or aboard a ship in U.S. territorial waters may be paid for by Medicare.

Part B: Medical Insurance

Part B medical insurance helps pay doctor bills, including those billed by affiliated HMOs; outpatient services; some home health care; and certain other medical services. *(See "Medicare at a Glance" on page 35.)*

It would be impossible to list, much less anticipate, the types of health care covered under Part B. We can make some generalizations, however. First, keep in mind that there is an annual deductible. In 2004 you will pay the first $100 of "allowable" charges per year. After that, you are responsible for paying 20 percent of all covered charges, plus any additional amount that a physician is allowed to charge. (A physician is prohibited from charging you more than 15 percent above the allowable charge.)

Example: Let's say that CMS sets an "allowable" charge for a particular health care service at $150. Your doctor does not have an agreement with Medicare to use CMS' rate schedule. If your doctor charges the maximum that Medicare will permit, he cannot bill you for more than $172.50, which is 115 percent of the "allowable" charge of $150.

Medicare Part B provides coverage for the services provided to you on an outpatient basis and for most supplies associated with those services. This includes coverage for physical therapy and speech pathology by doctors and institutional providers. Independent therapists are also given limited coverage under Part B insurance, based on certain dollar amounts per year. In addition, you'll be covered for certain nonroutine vision care provided by a qualified optometrist if it would have been covered by a physician. Also covered are diagnostic X-rays, lab tests and certain radiographic therapy treatments. (In fact, Medicare pays 100 percent of your diagnostic lab tests, rather than the 80 percent that applies to most tests.)

Covered Expenses

The following are common questions asked about covered expenses, some of which involve both Part A and Part B of Medicare.

Q. Are drugs and medicines covered under Medicare?

A. Generally, Medicare does not currently cover outpatient prescription drugs; however, there are several exceptions, such as non-self-administrable drugs provided as part of a physician's services, certain oral cancer drugs and erythropoietin for home dialysis patients. Medicare does help pay for the following items, but the coverage is limited for some:

- Antigens
- Hemophilia clotting factors
- Hepatitis B vaccine
- Immunosuppressive drugs
- Oral cancer drugs

Medicare Part A will pay for prescription drugs when you are in a hospital or a skilled nursing home and, on a more limited basis, when you are a hospice patient. Part B pays 80 percent of allowable charges for immunosuppressive drugs during the first year following a covered organ transplant (after the $100 annual deductible has been satisfied).

Note: As mentioned, Medicare will offer a voluntary drug benefit in 2006 and drug discount cards in 2004 and 2005.

Q. What about flu shots, pneumonia shots and hepatitis B vaccines?

A. Part B will also pay 100 percent of the approved charges for influenza (flu) and pneumococcal pneumonia vaccines and their administration (no deductible applies). If the person giving you the shot accepts "assignment" (accepts the Medicare payment as payment in full), there will be no charge to you. If the person doesn't accept assignment, you may have to pay charges in addition to the Medicare-approved amount (but not more than 15 percent over the approved charge).

CMS no longer requires that you have a physician write a prescription for flu or pneumonia shots given in a hospital, long-term care facility or by a home health agency.

If you are at medium to high risk for hepatitis B, Medicare will pay 80 percent of the Medicare-approved amount for the hepatitis B vaccination.

Q. What about coverage for blood or blood components?

A. Both Medicare hospital and medical insurance will help pay for blood (whole blood or units of packed red blood cells), blood components and the cost of blood processing and administration. You must pay any nonreplacement fees charged for the first three pints of whole blood or equivalent quantities of packed red blood cells you use each year, whether as an inpatient or outpatient.

You have the option of replacing the first three pints or units of blood on a pint-for-pint or unit basis, or paying the provider's customary charges for the unreplaced pints or units. You can either replace the blood personally or arrange to have another person or an organization replace it for you.

When you receive blood as a patient in a hospital or skilled nursing home, Medicare Part A may pay for blood processing (administration, storage, etc.), beginning with the first pint or unit in a calendar year. If you receive blood as an outpatient, you must replace or pay for the first three pints of blood and meet the $100 deductible before Medicare Part B helps pay. Part B will pay 80 percent of the approved amount for blood, starting with the fourth pint.

Note: If you've satisfied the nonreplacement fee charged for the first three units of blood under Medicare hospital insurance, you don't need to satisfy it again under Medicare medical insurance, and vice versa.

Q. Are ambulance services covered?

A. Medicare will cover transportation to a hospital, from a hospital to a skilled nursing facility or from a hospital or skilled nursing facility to your home. Medicare will also cover a round trip from a hospital or a participating skilled nursing facility to an outside supplier to obtain medically necessary diagnostic or therapeutic services not available where you are an inpatient.

Coverage is usually limited to transportation within your local area or to the nearest facility outside your area that can provide the necessary care. If there is a local facility equipped to provide the care you need but you choose to go to another institution farther away, Medicare's payment is based on the charge for transportation to the closest facility that can provide the necessary care. In addition to this restriction, Medicare Part B helps pay for medically necessary ambulance services only if:

- The ambulance, equipment and personnel meet Medicare requirements.
- Transportation in any other vehicle could endanger your health.

Medicare does not pay for ambulance transportation from your home to a doctor's office or to any free-standing facility, such as an ambulatory surgery center or a dialysis facility, that is not in or next to a hospital.

Medicare will pay for the use of an air ambulance only in extreme emergencies. If you could have been moved by land ambulance without seriously endangering your life, Medicare will pay only the land ambulance rate. You are responsible for the difference in costs.

Q. Will Medicare provide coverage for a wheelchair or other durable medical equipment?

A. Medicare will pay 80 percent of the cost of leasing, renting or buying a wheelchair and other durable medical equipment that your doctor prescribes for use in your home. To be considered durable medical equipment, the equipment must be able to withstand repeated use, primarily serve a medical purpose and be appropriate for home use.

Medicare pays for different kinds of durable medical equipment in various ways. Some equipment must be rented, other equipment must be purchased, and for some equipment you may choose rental or purchase. Your Medicare carrier will be able to provide more specific guidance on which method will be used for a particular item.

Before renting or purchasing equipment, prosthetics, orthotics or supplies, make sure that the supplier is Medicare-approved and has a Medicare supplier number. Medicare may not pay your claim if your supplier does not have this information. **Exception:** A supplier number is not necessary if the medical equipment or supplies are furnished incident to a physician's service.

Suppliers submit claims to one of four regional carriers for processing. Your supplier will need your permanent address to file your claim with the appropriate regional carrier. (Medicare considers your permanent residence to be the address where you intend to spend more than six months of the calendar year.)

The names and addresses of Medicare-participating suppliers are listed by geographical area in the *Medicare-Participating Supplier Directory*, which you can request by calling your durable medical equipment regional carrier. The directory also is available for your use at Social Security offices, state and area offices of the Administration on Aging and most hospitals, as well as online at ***www.medicare.gov***.

Caution: Medical equipment fraud continues to be a problem for Medicare beneficiaries. You should watch out for shady suppliers who may try to:

- Sell you unneeded or inappropriate equipment. Only your doctor should prescribe medical equipment for you.
- Promise you that items will be paid for by Medicare when, in fact, they are not eligible.
- Deliver defective products—or none at all.

If a supplier takes any of these actions, you should file a complaint with your Medicare carrier.

Q. Does Medicare pay for prosthetic devices?

A. There is some coverage: for example, for artificial limbs and eyes, corrective lenses needed after a cataract operation, ostomy bags and certain related supplies, breast prostheses after a mastectomy, and arm, leg, back and neck braces. Dental plates and other dental devices, however, are not covered.

Medicare does not pay for orthopedic shoes unless they are an integral part of leg braces and the cost is included in the charge for braces. Medicare does pay for therapeutic shoes and shoe inserts for people with severe diabetic foot disease.

Q. Are mammograms, pap smears and other screening tests covered?

A. Medicare pays 80 percent for annual mammograms for all Medicare-eligible women age 40 and older. Annual pap smears and pelvic exams are covered for Medicare enrollees at high risk while other women on Medicare are covered every third year. Medicare also helps pay for colorectal cancer screening for beneficiaries age 50 and older, bone density tests for women at high risk of osteoporosis and prostate cancer screenings for men age 50 and older. In 2005 screening for diabetes and heart disease will be added.

Q. What about mental health care?

A. Special payment rules apply to this kind of treatment. Medicare Part B helps pay for both partial hospitalization (also known as day treatment) services and nonhospital treatment of mental illnesses. Generally, you will have to pay one-half (rather than the usual 20 percent) of such outpatient charges, but your cost could be reduced to 20 percent if you would have required hospitalization without the outpatient treatment. This coverage includes services from doctors, physician assistants, psychologists, clinical social workers and comprehensive outpatient rehabilitation facilities (CORFs).

Note: CMS has instructed Medicare carriers not to deny claims automatically for patients diagnosed with Alzheimer's disease, which had been the policy in some cases. This means that Medicare may pay doctors and other health care professionals for diagnostic testing, medication management and psychological therapy for Alzheimer's patients.

Q. How is Medicare keeping up with advances in cancer treatment?

A. Medicare has recently expanded coverage of positron emission tomography (PET), an innovative imaging technology, to improve the care of patients with one of six types of cancer. It is also providing coverage for some patients with refractory epilepsy or who may be candidates for coronary revascularization.

PET usage may allow some Medicare beneficiaries to avoid undergoing invasive procedures and may provide information that will increase their confidence in the management of their care. CMS calls this development a major step toward broad cancer coverage.

Coverage Under Medicare and Veterans Benefits

If you are eligible for both Medicare and veterans benefits, you may choose to get treatment under either program. But Medicare (1) cannot pay for services you receive from veterans hospitals or other VA facilities, except for certain emergency hospital services or (2) generally cannot pay if the VA pays for VA-authorized services that you receive in a non-VA hospital or from a non-VA physician.

If you have coverage under a VA program (including CHAMPUS and CHAMPVA), your health benefits may change or end when you become eligible for Medicare. You should contact the Department of Veterans Affairs, Department of Defense or a military health benefits adviser for information before you decide whether to enroll in Medicare.

Some veterans who have nonservice-connected conditions and are above a certain income level are charged a VA co-payment for treatment in a VA hospital or medical facility or for VA-authorized treatment by non-VA sources. If the VA charges you a co-payment for VA-authorized care by a non-VA physician or hospital, Medicare may be able to reimburse you, in whole or in part, for your VA co-payment obligation. (If you have Medigap insurance, your Medigap policy may pay the VA co-insurance and deductible obligations, even if Medicare cannot.)

Q. Is it true that HMOs provide extra services that Medicare does not ordinarily cover?

A. Yes. Most HMOs and other prepaid health care organizations that enroll Medicare beneficiaries are required by law to provide, at no extra charge, some benefits that aren't available under traditional fee-for-service Medicare. These include extended stays in hospitals and skilled nursing facilities, expanded home health benefits, respite care and coverage for certain drugs. Also, many of these organizations offer, at little or no additional cost, services beyond those that Medicare covers, such as preventive care, dental care, hearing aids and eyeglasses.

Note: To receive Medicare coverage through an HMO or other prepaid health care plan, you must be enrolled in Medicare Part B and continue to pay the premiums. Also, you will usually be required to receive all care from your HMO, except in emergencies. *(For more information on HMOs, see Sections 4 and 5.)*

Q. Can I get extra services anywhere else?

A. Yes. Any Medicare beneficiary may seek the services offered through federally qualified health centers, which are located in both urban and rural areas. Medicare will help pay for services provided by these centers' physicians, nurse practitioners, clinical psychologists and other health care professionals. To help support these health centers, Medicare will also help pay for some preventive services that it otherwise would not cover. An added benefit is that you do not have to pay the annual Part B deductible for services provided by federally qualified health centers.

Items Not Covered by Medicare

Medicare has many exclusions. The simplest way to determine if an item is covered is to call your insurance carrier. Clearly, however, it does not cover some items, such as:

- Any health care service that you receive from a family member.
- Custodial care.
- Most prescription drugs taken at home (until 2006).
- Most immunizations.
- Self-administered injections, such as insulin.
- Routine physical examinations.
- Routine eye examinations.
- Dental care.
- Eyeglasses.
- Routine foot care (except for diabetics).
- Hearing aids.
- Cosmetic surgery (except following an accident).
- Private-duty nurses.
- Private hospital rooms (unless deemed necessary)
- TVs and telephones in a hospital.
- Orthopedic shoes.

Exception: Medicare will help pay for therapeutic shoes and shoe inserts—one pair per calendar year—for those who have severe diabetic foot disease, as long as a physician certifies the need and supplies are prescribed by a podiatrist and furnished by a podiatrist, an orthotist or a prosthetist.

Q. How can I get information about coverage for kidney failure?

A. Call the Medicare hotline at (800) 633-4227 and ask for Publication 610A, *Medicare Coverage of Kidney Dialysis and Kidney Transplant Services*, or view it online at *www.medicare.gov*.

Q. What is a Medicare Summary Notice?

A. This is an easy-to-read monthly statement that spells out your health insurance claims information. You should read these notices carefully to make sure you have received the services, medical equipment and supplies for which Medicare was billed. If you disagree with a claims decision, you may appeal by following the instructions on the notice.

Remember: Your Medicare Summary Notice is not a bill. Always wait until you receive a bill before sending any money to a health care provider.

Q. Will Medicare pay for second opinions before surgery?

A. Medicare encourages and will help pay for a second opinion before non-emergency surgery. Your own doctor can refer you to another, or you can call your Medicare insurance carrier for references. If the first and second opinions are contradictory, Medicare will help pay for a third opinion.

3

Medicare Costs and Claims

Medicare isn't free. In most cases you will share the costs of Medicare through six types of payments: premiums, deductibles, co-payments, extended care, fees for drugs or medicines and the deductible for receiving blood. Qualified Social Security recipients do not have to pay for Part A insurance; they do have to pay a monthly premium for Part B, just as they do for any other insurance policy.

Q. How much will Medicare cost me?

A. In 2004 the least expensive monthly premium for Part B medical insurance is $66.60 if you enroll at the earliest opportunity. Delaying enrollment may result in a higher premium. Similarly, if you enroll and then drop out only to re-enroll later, your premiums may also be higher. Basically, you will pay an additional charge of 10 percent for every 12 months that you did not participate when you could have done so. The premium you pay is automatically deducted from your monthly Social Security check and is adjusted each Jan. 1. The government sets the premium amounts annually according to statutory formulas.

Q. What are the deductibles?

A. These are the initial expenses you have to pay before Medicare starts to pick up any costs. Under Part A, if you are hospitalized in 2004, you will pay for the first $876 of treatment in each benefit period. A benefit period ends 60 days after your discharge from either a hospital or a skilled nursing facility. If you're hospitalized after that, you will have to pay another deductible, as well as the various other cost-sharing amounts.

Under Part B medical insurance, the deductible is currently $100 per year of the charges *allowable* by Medicare. If you are charged an additional fee for a service that is not considered allowable, you will have to pay for that charge, too, unless you successfully protest the fee.

Co-Payments: Paying Your Share

Co-payments, also called co-insurance, represent your share of health care costs. Whether or not you will have to make co-payments depends on the kind of care provided and where you received it.

Q. Are there co-payments for hospitalization?

A. There are no co-payments for hospital stays of 60 days or less. All approved hospital costs are picked up by Medicare for the first 60 days, once you have paid the deductible in each benefit period ($876 in 2004). You must pay for personal conveniences, such as the extra cost of a private room (unless medically necessary), TV rental, telephone and private-duty nurses.

However, after 60 days of hospitalization, you will have to pay an additional charge of $219 per day. If you are still hospitalized after 90 days, there are additional costs—as well as a choice: Either you can pay $438 per day for up to 60 (nonrenewable) "lifetime reserve" days, or you can pay the full amount of the charges yourself. Hospitals will assume that you want to use your lifetime reserve days unless you specify otherwise in writing (either when you are admitted to the hospital or up to 90 days after you are discharged).

Note: If you use reserve days and then decide that you did not want to do so, you must request approval from the hospital to get them restored.

If you are out of the hospital for at least 60 days in a row and then are readmitted, a new benefit period begins—that is, your 90 days of coverage start all over again. You will also have to pay the deductible amount again.

Q. How do co-payments apply for other inpatient care?

A. For care in a skilled nursing facility, Medicare hospital insurance helps pay for up to 100 days per benefit period once you are admitted to a skilled care facility. Medicare pays all approved costs for the first 20 days. In 2004 you will pay $109.50 a day thereafter (rates are adjusted annually), for a possible total of $8,760, should you have to stay for a full 100 days. Again, you have to pay for personal items such as TV rental, private nurses, a private room (unless medically necessary) and custodial services (help with eating, dressing, etc.). Prescription drugs furnished by the facility during your stay are covered, just as they would be in a hospital.

If you leave a skilled nursing facility and are readmitted within 30 days for further treatment of the same condition, you do not need to have a new three-day hospital stay to qualify for coverage, provided that you have some of your 100 days left. After 100 days, if you don't have a long-term-care insurance policy, you will have to pay for the stay yourself.

Certain home health care—such as physical therapy, part-time skilled nursing and medical supplies—may be paid for in full by Medicare when you are confined at home under care specifically prescribed by your doctor. Make sure that you contract for such services with a home health agency that participates in Medicare.

For hospice care, five days of respite care in a hospice (to assist your primary caretaker) can be covered up to 95 percent by Medicare. The patient is responsible for paying 5 percent of the cost of outpatient drugs, up to a maximum of $5 per prescription.

For care in psychiatric hospitals, a lifetime 190-day limitation for inpatient psychiatric care applies. Further restrictions apply if you are already hospitalized as a psychiatric inpatient when you are first covered by Medicare.

Q. How do co-payments apply to doctors' services and to other outpatient services?

A. Under Part B of your Medicare insurance, after paying your $100 deductible, you will be responsible for 20 percent of all remaining approved charges (with the exception of mental health service charges, which might be as high as 50 percent). Medicare pays 80 percent of all approved charges, once you have met your $100 annual deductible. For example, if your doctor charges an approved rate of $75 for a visit, Medicare will pay $60 and you will pay $15, once you have satisfied the deductible for that benefit period.

If your physician charges more than the Medicare-approved amount for any given service, you will likely have to pay both the co-payment for the Medicare-approved amount and the excess over that amount, up to the ceiling of 115 percent that Medicare calls the "limiting charge." In a few instances Medicare will pay 100 percent of all Part B costs, such as for clinical diagnostic laboratory tests. (To find out what the limiting charge is for a particular service, you should contact your Medicare carrier. Limiting-charge information will also appear on your Medicare Summary Notice when you receive medical services covered by Medicare.)

If you are disabled and return to work, you will be allowed to retain your Part A coverage premium-free for up to 8½ years.

Medicare and Physicians

Medicare coverage is restricted to services provided by licensed medical doctors and osteopaths. Other practitioners who can furnish some covered services include chiropractors, podiatrists, optometrists, dentists and dental surgeons.

The only chiropractic service Medicare covers is for manual manipulation of the spine to correct a subluxation (a partial dislocation), which must be indicated on an X-ray.

Q. How do I find a doctor who accepts Medicare patients?

A. To locate physicians in your area, check the *Medicare-Participating Physician/Supplier Directory*, available free from your Medicare carrier or online at *www.medicare.gov*. You can also find copies at your local Social Security office, your state Agency on Aging and most hospitals.

Physicians and suppliers are given the opportunity each year to sign participation agreements. To find out if a certain doctor participates in Medicare, call his office and ask. Or look for the red and gray emblem in his office that says "Accepts Assignment on All Medicare Claims." Remember, a nonparticipating physician can accept assignment for one claim and refuse to accept it for another. You can always ask your doctor if he will accept assignment before you agree to a specific treatment.

Q. Does anyone rate the doctors who participate in Medicare?

A. No single group or agency rates physicians. Your best bet for a recommendation is probably a satisfied patient. Check with other Medicare beneficiaries in your area to see which doctors they prefer and why.

Q. What if my physician does not participate in Medicare?

A. If you go to a nonparticipating physician—one who has not signed an agreement with CMS to take "assignment" (that is, to accept the Medicare-approved fee as total payment for her services)—you will have to foot the bill for any difference between the Medicare-approved amount and the limiting charge. Any doctor can accept Medicare payments, so be sure to ask your doctor if she will do so. If not, ask the doctor to refer you to a participating Medicare physician.

Q. What is the "limiting charge"?

A. This is the highest fee a nonparticipating physician can charge a Medicare patient for a covered service. Currently, the limiting charge is 115 percent of the approved amount. If your bill was $115 and the approved amount $100, Medicare would pay $80 and you would pay $35 (the $20 co-payment plus the $15 difference between the approved amount and the physician's fee), provided you had already satisfied the annual deductible.

Q. What if my physician charges more than the limiting charge?

A. You don't have to pay it. It is illegal for nonparticipating doctors to charge Medicare patients more than the approved amount plus 15 percent. Moreover, all physicians and qualified laboratories must accept the Medicare-approved amount as full payment for Medicare-covered clinical diagnostic laboratory tests.

Q. How will I know if I have been overcharged?

A. Most Medicare payments are based on fee schedules, which vary by region and physician specialty. Medicare fee schedules list the approved payment for each covered service. When a claim is submitted, your carrier compares the actual charge with the amount on the fee schedule and pays whichever is lower. Medicare follows up by sending you a Medicare Summary Notice. It shows what services were covered and what charges were approved, including the limiting charges for the services performed.

Q. What can I do if I've been overcharged?

A. Talk to your doctor first. If you can't resolve the problem together, call or write to your Medicare carrier.

Q. Do I have to pay for tests my doctor ordered that are not covered by Medicare?

A. That depends. Your doctor must give you a written notice if she knows or believes that Medicare will consider a service medically unreasonable and unnecessary and therefore won't pay for it. If your doctor gave you such a notice and you signed an agreement to pay for the service yourself, you are responsible for paying for it. If your doctor did not give you a written notice, however, and you did not know the service wasn't covered, you cannot be held liable to pay.

Note: The doctor's written notice is not an official determination by Medicare. Your doctor can submit a claim on your behalf. If Medicare rejects it, you can appeal its decision. You have six months from the date of the decision to ask your carrier to review it. If the carrier turns you down and the amount in question is $100 or more, you can continue to appeal. Cases involving $1,000 or more can eventually be appealed to a federal court.

Handling Claims

Hospital and medical claims are handled differently. By law, the only items for which a participating hospital or health care facility can bill you are the applicable deductible and co-insurance amounts, as well as noncovered items such as TV rental, private nurses and custodial care. The law requires participating hospitals and skilled nursing facilities to accept Medicare payments as payment in full for covered services. The hospital or nursing home will bill you directly for any services rendered after your coverage ends.

In terms of medical claims, all doctors and suppliers are now required to fill out and send in Medicare claim forms for you, even if they don't take assignment (that is, accept the amount approved by Medicare as total payment for their services). Doctors, suppliers and other providers of Part B services have one year from the date of your service to send in your claim. Your doctor or supplier cannot escape the obligation to submit a claim by requiring you to sign an agreement that no claim will be submitted. In some cases, you may need to file your own Medicare Part B claim.

➤ **Recommendation:** If you have other health insurance that should pay before Medicare, you can—and should—submit the claims yourself.

Q. If the doctor takes assignment, will I still get a bill?

A. Yes. You will be billed by your Medicare insurance carrier for any part of the $100 annual deductible you still owe, as well as for the co-insurance amount (20 percent) and for services Medicare doesn't cover, such as routine checkups.

Medicare Coverage at a Glance—Part A Hospital Insurance Services (Premium-Free for Most Recipients)

Services	Benefit	Medicare Pays	You Pay*
Hospitalization Semiprivate room and board, general nursing and other hospital services and supplies	First 60 days	All but $876	$876
	61st to 90th day	All but $219 a day	$219 a day
	91st to 150th day	All but $438 a day	$438 a day
	Beyond 150 days**	Nothing	All costs
Skilled Nursing Facility*** Semiprivate room and board, skilled nursing and rehabilitative services and other services and supplies	First 20 days	100% of approved amount	Nothing
	Additional 80 days	All but $109.50 a day	Up to $109.50 a day
	Beyond 100 days	Nothing	All costs
Home Health Care Intermittent skilled care, home health aide services, durable medical equipment and supplies and other services	Unlimited as long as you meet Medicare conditions	100% of approved amount; 80% of approved amount for durable medical equipment	Nothing for services; 20% of approved amount for durable medical equipment
Hospice Care Pain relief, symptom management and support services for the terminally ill	As long as doctor certifies need	All but limited cost for outpatient drugs and inpatient respite care	Limited costs for outpatient drugs and inpatient respite care
Blood**** When furnished by a hospital or skilled nursing facility during a covered stay	Unlimited if medically necessary	All but first 3 pints per calendar year	For first 3 pints

Part A monthly premium for 2004 is free for most beneficiaries. For beneficiaries who worked fewer than 30 quarters, the premium is $343; for those who worked between 30 and 40 quarters, the premium is $189.

*For calendar year 2004, per benefit period, subject to change each Jan. 1.

**Each beneficiary has 60 reserve days that can be used only once in a lifetime.

***Medicare will not pay for most nursing home care or custodial care, also called long-term care.

****If you've paid for blood under Part B, you need not pay again under Part A.

Medicare Coverage at a Glance—Part B Medical Insurance Services (Basic Monthly Premium: $66.60*)

Services	Benefit	Medicare Pays	You Pay**
Medical Expenses Doctors' services, outpatient medical and surgical services and supplies, outpatient physical and speech therapy, diagnostic tests, durable medical equipment and other services	Unlimited if medically necessary	80% of approved amount (after $100 annual deductible); reduced to 50% for most outpatient mental health services	$100 annual deductible, plus 20% of approved amount (and limited charges above approved amount)
Clinical Laboratory Services Blood tests, urinalyses, etc.	Unlimited if medically necessary	Generally 100% of approved amount	Nothing for services
Home Health Care Intermittent skilled care, home health aide services, durable medical equipment and supplies and other services	Unlimited as long as you meet Medicare conditions	100% of amount; 80% of approved amount for durable medical equipment	Nothing for services; 20% of approved amount for durable medical equipment
Outpatient Hospital Treatment Services for diagnosis or treatment of illness or injury	Unlimited if medically necessary	Medicare payment to hospital based on reasonable cost	20% of billed amount (after $100 annual deductible)
Blood* **	Unlimited if medically necessary	80% of approved amount (after $100 deductible and starting with 4th pint)	For first 3 pints plus 20% of approved amount for additional pints (after $100 deductible)

*For 2004 (premium may be higher if you enroll late); subject to change each Jan. 1.

**You pay the $100 deductible only once per calendar year, whatever combination of services you use.

***If you've paid for blood under Part A, you need not pay again under Part B.

Claims for Deceased Patients

When a Medicare beneficiary dies, the way Medicare pays Part B claims depends on whether the doctor's or supplier's bill has been paid. (Any Part A payments due to the hospital, skilled nursing facility, home health agency or hospice will be made directly to the provider of services.)

If the bill was paid by the patient or with funds from the patient's estate, Medicare's payment will be made either to the estate representative or to a surviving member of the patient's immediate family. If someone other than the patient paid the bill, payment may be made to that person.

If the bill has not been paid and the doctor or supplier does not accept assignment, the Medicare payment can be made to the person who has or assumes the legal obligation to pay the bill for the deceased patient. Your Medicare carrier can provide additional information about how to claim a Medicare Part B payment after a patient dies.

Q. Do I have to pay the bill before my doctor submits it?

A. That's up to your doctor. If she accepts assignment, you need not pay in advance. In all cases, your claims will be submitted by the provider.

Q. How will I know what Medicare has covered and what I still owe?

A. Medicare sends you a Medicare Summary Notice after it reviews your claim. It shows what services were covered, what charges it will pay and what you are responsible for paying. If it's a Part B claim, it also shows how much was credited toward your $100 annual deductible.

Q. What if I don't agree with a payment decision?

A. You have the right to appeal. The notice explaining benefits tells you what steps you can take. Or you can call Social Security, the insurance intermediary, the carrier handling the claim for Medicare or your state's PRO.

Q. What if I have other insurance as well? Where do I file my claim?

A. File first with the non-Medicare insurer in any of the following situations:

- You are still working and are covered by an employer group health plan.
- You are disabled, are under age 65 and are covered under an employer's health plan.
- You have a work-related illness or injury. Workers' compensation should cover the services that are provided to treat the work-related illness or injury.

4

Additional Coverage

As you can see from the issues raised in the previous sections, Medicare's traditional fee-for-service coverage is far from comprehensive. You will need to develop a strategy to avoid exposure to steep health care bills. What approaches should you consider?

If you're still working, you might be able to rely on your employer's health plan; some companies provide coverage for retirees as well. Another option is to blend some form of private insurance that you purchase yourself with traditional Medicare coverage. In recent years, many Medicare enrollees have opted for managed care—prepaid comprehensive health plans. In this section we will examine and compare these different systems.

Employer-Provided Insurance

This type of insurance is usually available to those who are employed and in some cases also to retirees. If you continue to work after 65, regulations mandate that employees and their spouses be offered the opportunity to remain in their company health plans. (Currently, this rule applies to companies with 20 or more employees.)

If you (or your spouse) continue to work after age 65 and accept an employer's health plan, it becomes your primary insurance. In that case, the company's insurance carrier is billed first, and Medicare picks up the remaining eligible costs. Whether you will want to enroll in or keep Medicare medical insurance depends on how fully the plan offered through your employer or former employer covers doctors' bills and other health services that Medicare covers. In other words, you will need to consider whether Medicare's secondary benefits are worth the cost. This means you're going to have to compare what you can afford against what is offered.

➤ **Observation:** Remember, you do not have to enroll in Medicare medical insurance (Part B) to get premium-free Medicare hospital insurance (Part A).

If you are retired and are covered by an employer's retiree benefit plan, Medicare is your primary payer. But if you make that choice, the employer's plan is not permitted to pay supplemental benefits for Medicare-covered services. It is permitted, though, to offer a plan that pays for services not covered by Medicare, such as hearing aids and routine dental care.

Special rules apply

When you have health insurance from an employer group health plan, there are some special rules to keep in mind.

For those age 65 or older: If you (or your spouse) continue to work and are covered under an employer group health plan, you can wait to enroll in Medicare medical insurance during a seven-month "special enrollment period." This period begins with the month that the group health coverage ends, or the month that employment ends—whichever comes first. If you meet certain requirements, you won't have to wait for a general enrollment period, and you won't have to pay the 10 percent premium surcharge for late enrollment in Medicare.

In the event that you reject the employer's health plan, Medicare will be your primary health insurance payer. The employer is not allowed to offer you Medicare supplemental coverage if you reject the company's health plan.

For those under age 65: If you (or another family member) are employed and you have health coverage under a "large group health plan," Medicare will be the secondary payer. A large group health plan covers employees of a firm or group of firms where at least one firm has 100 or more workers. In that case, you will also have the special enrollment period and premium rights that are available to workers age 65 or older.

What happens if you are under age 65, entitled to Medicare because of permanent kidney failure and have employer group health coverage? Medicare will be the secondary payer for the first 18 months of your Medicare Part A (hospital insurance) eligibility. At the end of the 18-month period, Medicare becomes your primary payer.

➤ **Recommendation:** If you are not sure whether any of these rules applies to you, call your local Social Security office. If you have questions about the size of your group health plan, check with your employer's personnel office.

Before you retire, check your employer's health insurance policy to see if it offers you the option of continuing your coverage. If so, examine the benefits to see if they cover some or most of the gaps in Medicare coverage outlined in previous sections. Consult your company's benefits counselor. Be sure to follow up all conversations with written memoranda confirming your understanding.

Once you're retired, Medicare will usually be your primary carrier. So if the benefits available from your employer's plan are similar to those offered by "Medigap" policies (which are specifically designed to supplement Medicare benefits, as noted later in this section), it will probably be worth continuing your coverage. Note that one major advantage of continuing with your employer's plan is that you don't have to wait to be covered for pre-existing conditions.

Caution: The IRS, CMS and the SSA share information about whether Medicare beneficiaries or their spouses are working and whether they have employment-related health insurance. The process, known as Data Match, helps Medicare find cases where another insurer should pay first on Medicare beneficiaries' health care claims. CMS also gets information about which insurer should pay first through the Initial Enrollment Questionnaire that you receive after enrolling in Medicare but before coverage takes effect. If you believe that CMS' information about your other health insurance is incorrect, call your insurance carrier.

There are other special situations in which Medicare is not always the primary payer. For example, Medicare may be the secondary payer if you are entitled to veterans benefits, workers' compensation or black-lung benefits. It can also be the secondary payer if no-fault insurance or liability insurance (such as automobile insurance) is available as the primary payer. For more details on this subject, refer to the publication *Medicare Secondary Payer*, which is available from any Social Security office or online at ***www.medicare.gov***.

Managed-Care Plans

In a managed-care plan, such as a health maintenance organization (HMO), a network of health care providers (doctors, hospitals, skilled nursing facilities and so forth) generally offers comprehensive, coordinated medical services to plan members on a prepaid basis. Depending on how the plan is organized, care is provided at a central facility or in the private-practice offices of the doctors and other professionals affiliated with the plan.

In 1998 the government granted sweeping protections to Medicare beneficiaries that contained special provisions for managed-care plans. Among the federal regulations:

- No one can be denied enrollment in a health plan on account of mental or physical illness, genetic information, disability or prior use of medical care.
- Women can demand "direct access to a women's health specialist" for routine and preventive health care services.
- A general health assessment must be performed within 90 days of enrollment in any managed-care plan. If a medical condition exists, a treatment protocol must be developed and implemented.

Most managed-care plans provide preventive health care and other services that are not covered by Medicare, such as routine physicals, health education and dental care. Some offer vision care; many provide some coverage for prescription drugs—a major concern for many Medicare beneficiaries.

Depending on your perspective, one plus or minus of prepaid plans is that they offer a single network of care. You are able to select a primary care physician from among those in the managed-care plan, but if you require a specialist or hospitalization, the plan will decide whom you will see. The costs, however, are predictable, which can be a real advantage for retirees on a fixed income.

If you enroll in a managed-care plan, Medicare makes a payment to the plan to provide you with all the services covered by Medicare. In addition, the plan may charge you a nominal co-payment at the time of service; most charge a monthly premium in place of the usual Medicare co-insurance and deductibles. (Remember: You are still responsible for payment of your Medicare Part B premium. If you receive a monthly Social Security check, the premium is withheld from your check. This obligation is separate from your payment to the plan.) The plan may also offer you expanded coverage at a higher premium. In some cases, the expanded coverage is optional, but in others, it is an enrollment requirement.

Lock-in provisions

Although as a plan member you are generally "locked in" to receiving care from the plan's providers, the lock-in does not apply to the following:

- Emergency services, which you may receive anywhere.
- Urgently needed care, which you may receive while you are temporarily away from the plan's service area.
- Services provided by a nonplan health care provider to whom the plan referred you.

If you join a plan with a lock-in provision, this will be explained in your membership packet, which includes a list of the plan's health care providers. You will also receive a letter from the Medicare program explaining the lock-in provision and confirming your enrollment in the plan.

If you enroll in a plan that does not have a lock-in requirement, you can use nonplan health care professionals. Although the plan generally will not pay if you use nonplan providers, Medicare will still pay its share for covered expenses. In such instances, you would be responsible for paying Medicare's co-insurance, deductibles and other permissible charges, just as if you were receiving care under the traditional fee-for-service system.

Enrollment period

All HMOs have an advertised open enrollment period at least annually for a minimum of 30 days. You can join during any open enrollment period and stay with the plan as long as you like. Depending on the plan, coverage can begin either on the first day of the month after the plan receives your enrollment application or up to three months later.

➤ **Recommendation:** If you discover that your bills for Medicare services are not being paid because you recently joined a plan or changed plans, contact your local Social Security office. If your plan refuses to pay for or provide a Medicare-covered service, you may make a written appeal to the plan. Under federal law, a plan must respond within 14 days (within three days if a life-threatening condition is involved). The information provided when you joined a plan will explain your appeal rights.

What if you decide you want to stop your HMO coverage? Send a signed request to your HMO or your local Social Security (or Railroad Retirement Board) office. Note that if you disenroll from a managed-care plan, your coverage under fee-for-service Medicare will begin on the first day of the following month. Medicare HMO members who want to switch back to a traditional fee-for-service approach may be turned down for Medigap coverage *(see page 45)* if they have health problems, or they might have to pay higher premiums.

Caution: It's important to choose a plan carefully. Under current regulations, you will be able to change plans only once, between Jan. 1 and March 31, and will be locked in for the rest of the year.

Care outside your service area

If you move away from the plan's service area or you intend to be away from the area for more than 90 days at a time, you must notify the plan. Generally, you will be disenrolled from the plan if you have moved permanently or the absence lasts longer than 90 days. Plans are permitted to retain members who are temporarily absent from the plan's service area, but some restrictions may apply.

If you travel frequently, you should consider several factors before deciding whether to join a managed-care plan. For example, a plan member who is temporarily away from the plan's service area is not entitled to coverage of any care other than emergency or urgently needed services. If you have a medical emergency, you can see a local doctor or go to a nearby hospital. Your Medicare HMO will pay the provider who treats you. Your maximum out-of-pocket cost is limited to the lesser of $50 or the fee the plan would have charged. Some Medicare HMOs have arrangements with HMOs in other areas to provide out-of-area coverage. (Treatment outside the United States is not usually covered.)

If you're dropped from your HMO . . .

Under certain circumstances a Medicare managed-care plan can disenroll you without your permission. Before the HMO does so, however, it must attempt to contact you regarding the reason for its action and then send you a written notice. You will be given the opportunity to respond to the notice before the disenrollment takes effect.

You may be disenrolled from your plan for any of the following reasons:

- You discontinue your Medicare Part B coverage.
- You fail to pay premiums or approved co-payments charged by the plan, and the plan has given you a reasonable chance to make the payments.
- You move out of the plan's service area, or you leave the area for more than 90 consecutive days. (You can choose to join a Medicare health plan in your new area.)
- You commit fraud or allow someone else to use your membership card.

- Your behavior is disruptive, unruly, abusive or uncooperative to the extent that your continuing membership seriously impairs the plan's ability to furnish services to you or to other members. (CMS must approve this action.)
- The plan's Medicare contract is canceled or is not renewed. In either case, you will be given the opportunity to enroll in another plan (if there's one in the area) or to return to traditional fee-for-service Medicare. The plan must notify you at least 60 days before the end of the contract and, if necessary, must arrange for coverage of pre-existing conditions if you choose to buy a Medigap policy.

If you're dropped from a Medicare HMO, take the following steps:

- **Stay with your HMO until the last possible date.** If you drop out sooner, your withdrawal will be considered "voluntary" and you will forfeit certain guarantees of future coverage.
- **Check into alternatives right away** so that you'll be ready to change plans when your HMO shuts its doors to Medicare enrollees.
- **Consider switching from managed care** to traditional Medicare with a Medigap policy *(see page 45)*. If you don't withdraw prematurely, you're guaranteed the opportunity to buy Medigap Plan A, B, C or F, regardless of your health *(see chart on page 47)*. This option allows you to choose your own doctors, including specialists.

To use the guarantees above, you must act within 63 days. That is, if your Medicare HMO coverage ends on Dec. 31, your right to buy one of the four Medigap policies expires on the following March 5.

- **Shop carefully for Medigap policies** because prices vary widely. For example, a 65-year-old woman in Connecticut could pay anywhere from $1,622 to $2,456 per year for a Medigap Plan F, according to Weiss Ratings of Palm Beach Gardens, Fla.
- **Check on future price increases.** Some Medigap policies are inexpensive initially but automatically increase your premiums as your grow older.
- **If you can't afford a Medigap policy,** seek a replacement HMO. Be aware, though, that your new HMO might bail out of Medicare at some future date.

Look for accreditation

More employers are insisting that their managed-care providers submit to accreditation. The National Committee for Quality Assurance (NCQA), based in Washington, D.C., is one of the external accreditation review groups emerging to meet this need.

The NCQA evaluates HMOs and preferred provider organizations (PPOs). It requires that managed-care organizations meet or exceed 50 quality benchmarks or tests of quality improvement. The areas tested include doctors' credentials, pre-

HMO Enrollment Criteria

HMOs cannot screen their applicants to find out how healthy they are or delay coverage for pre-existing conditions. The only enrollment criteria for Medicare beneficiaries are:

- You must be enrolled in Medicare Part B (medical insurance) and continue to pay Part B premiums.
- You must live in the plan's service area.
- You cannot be receiving care in a Medicare-certified hospice.
- They will not accept people with permanent kidney failure. **Exception:** If you are a member of a managed-care plan when you first become eligible for Medicare and the plan has a Medicare contract, you may change to Medicare membership with the plan even if you have end-stage renal disease.

ventive health services, utilization management, medical records and the rights and responsibilities of members. Additionally, some states, such as Florida and Pennsylvania, are requiring outside evaluations of managed-care providers that do business within their boundaries.

When it comes to patient satisfaction, there may be vast differences among Medicare HMOs, which now have to make their dropout rates available to the public. (The government mails Medicare participants a list of plans in their area, along with information on benefits, costs and quality.) At the very least, you should be cautious about plans where the dropout rate exceeds the 15 percent national average—that's a sign of consumer unhappiness.

Despite all the negative publicity about HMOs, an NCQA study released in 2003 found that HMOs and POS plans reported promising trends for the fourth straight year in the face of rising health care costs. In 2002, for example, the percentage of women ages 21 to 64 who were screened for cervical cancer increased a notch over 2001 (to more than 80 percent); blood pressure control was up three points (to 57 percent); the percentage of people receiving a beta blocker after a heart attack topped 93 percent, "approaching the ideal" for this treatment.

Moreover, the average rates for key indicators of member satisfaction are also encouraging. The percentage of members who rated their health plan 8, 9 or 10 out of 10 increased from 59 percent in 2000 to 61 percent in 2002, according to the NCQA. Members expressed even greater satisfaction with customer service: 70 percent said they didn't encounter problems in obtaining plan information, getting help or completing paperwork (up from 54 percent as recently as 1998).

New 'social HMOs'

Medicare has begun to experiment with "social HMOs," which arrange for services such as housekeeping and home-delivered meals as well as medical care. Four plans already are in place, covering metro Los Angeles; Las Vegas and southern Nevada; Portland, Ore.; and New York City. Altogether, more than 100,000 people are enrolled.

If you're 65 and live in one of these areas, you can opt to join a social HMO when you apply for Medicare, even if you don't need its aging-in-place services right away. If you develop a chronic illness or become frail, the HMO will assign a "personal care planner" to arrange for medical, social and in-home services after receiving the approval of a case manager.

Such services aren't free, but they're less expensive than if you were to buy them on your own. For instance, at the Los Angeles social HMO, the co-payment for a home-delivered meal is $2; the cost is $8.50 per visit for transportation to medical or dental appointments, housekeeping services and help with bathing and dressing.

(For more details on Medicare HMOs, see Section 5.)

Other Types of Policies

Association group insurance

Many voluntary organizations offer group health coverage to members age 65 and older. Beware of advertisements of low rates, however, because this coverage can actually cost more than comparable individual policies. Be sure you understand the benefits offered, and then compare prices. Ask for written explanations of benefits and concerns, and be wary of any organization that refuses to provide a written explanation.

Private insurance

If the three group alternatives above (employer-provided insurance, managed-care plans and association insurance) don't provide the type of coverage you need, you might consider an individual health insurance policy. There are a large number of private health care policies for people 65 and older, including Medigap and long-term-care policies. They range from sound financial investments to outright scams.

Hospital indemnity policies

These plans pay a fixed amount for each day you spend in a hospital, up to a specified limit. Some also pay a fixed amount for surgery or for days spent in a skilled nursing home. Hospital indemnity policies generally pay the specified benefit regardless of your other health coverage. While Medicare hospital insurance covers most of your hospital costs, some people find that cash from an indemnity policy helps them with other expenses associated with illness or injury.

Be sure that any indemnity policy you buy allows benefits to increase periodically in line with hospital costs. Many consumer advocates advise Medicare participants to be particularly cautious when considering these policies because they tend to be superfluous.

Specified-disease insurance

This type of insurance, which is not available in every state, provides benefits only if you contract a given disease, such as cancer, or a group of specified diseases. Benefits are usually limited to payment of a fixed amount for each type of treatment. The value of such coverage depends on your chances of contracting the disease. Unless you have a crystal ball with special powers of divining the future, you are likely to find it a waste of money.

Note: Medicare and any additional insurance policy you have, such as a standard Medigap policy, will probably cover the costs associated with any of the specified diseases you might contract.

Travel policies

Medicare generally does not pay for hospitalization or medical services rendered outside the United States, as noted in Section 2. Yet because so many people travel today, medical coverage in a foreign country is increasingly important. For example, some insurers offer special short-term health insurance for foreign travel. Such plans are offered by several companies, including Access America, (800) 284-8300; Travel Guard, (800) 782-5151; and Wallach and Company, (800) 237-6615.

Supplemental Medigap Policies

Medigap policies are supplemental policies that attempt to fill the gap created by Medicare's limits on coverage. They cover such items as deductibles, co-insurance amounts, charges for health care services and supplies not covered by Medicare, and the Medicare-eligible expenses you may incur after Medicare's limits have been reached. Medigap insurance is available only to those age 65 and older.

The first six months you are enrolled in Medicare Part B and are age 65 or older constitute your Medigap open enrollment period. If you apply during this period, the Medigap insurer cannot refuse to issue you a policy, cannot place conditions on the policy or discriminate in the price of the policy because of your health status, claims experience, history of health care usage or your medical condition.

Note: Your Medigap open enrollment period is a one-time opportunity. After the six-month period, you may not be able to buy the Medigap policy of your choice at the best price.

For many years, the proliferation of these policies made it difficult to tell the good from the bad. In 1990 Congress passed legislation attempting to unify and simplify the coverage that could be offered. As a result, Medicare supplemental coverage is now limited to 10 standard plans, named "A" through "J," with "A" providing the basic or core supplemental coverage.

If you are under 65 and covered by a hospital or medical-expense policy, such as hospital-surgical, major medical or comprehensive health insurance, your coverage will probably end on your 65th birthday. But you may be given a chance to convert it to a Medigap policy. If you convert your old policy, you will be issued a new one by the same insurer, with benefits that complement those of Medicare. The advantage is that you need not wait for coverage of existing medical problems that have already been approved.

How Medigap works

The 10 basic Medigap policies offer varied levels of coverage, but not every insurer will offer every plan, and not all the plans may be available in every state. Each of the 10 policies (labeled "A" to "J") must offer the core benefits provided in policy "A." "B" through "J" offer various combinations of additional benefits *(see chart on next page)*. Insurers are not permitted to change the combination of benefits in any of the 10 standard plans.

A state may limit the number of plans available for sale to fewer than 10, but all states are required to allow the sale of the basic Plan A. To make it easier for consumers to compare plans and premiums, insurers must use the same format, language and definitions to describe the benefits of the 10 plans. Thus each company's products are alike, so the insurers are competing on reliability, service and price.

Plan "A" policies cover the following costs and services:

- The standard Part A co-insurance amounts for hospital care.
- Coverage for 100 percent of Medicare's Part A eligible hospital expenses after all Medicare benefits are exhausted, for up to a maximum of 365 days of additional inpatient hospital care during the policyholder's lifetime.
- The standard Part B co-insurance amounts for medical care.
- Patient's contribution for the first three units of blood or blood components not covered by Medicare Parts A and B.

Other standardized policies cover such items as:

- The co-insurance amount you would otherwise pay for skilled care in a nursing home from the 21st day to the 100th day of care ($109.50 per day in 2004).
- The Medicare Part A hospital deductible ($876 per benefit period in 2004).
- The Medicare Part B medical deductible ($100 per calendar year in 2004).
- Either 80 percent or 100 percent of excess physicians' fees and other Part B medical service charges, up to the limiting charge set by either Medicare or state law.
- Necessary emergency medical care in a foreign country. After you meet a $250 annual deductible, this benefit covers 80 percent of the costs of emergency medical care begun during the first two months of each trip outside the United States. There is a lifetime maximum cap of $50,000 on this benefit.
- At-home recovery. This benefit is being more strictly administered than in the past. Not only are fraud and abuse in home health care being investigated more vigorously, but there are more stringent requirements on the physician

The 10 Standard Medigap Plans

Coverage	A	B	C	D	E	F	G	H	I	J
Core benefits	✓	✓	✓	✓	✓	✓	✓	✓	✓	✓
Skilled nursing facility care			✓	✓	✓	✓	✓	✓	✓	✓
Hospital deductible		✓	✓	✓	✓	✓	✓	✓	✓	✓
Medical deductible			✓			✓				✓
Excess medical charges						100%	80%		100%	100%
Foreign treatment			80%	80%	80%	80%	80%	80%	80%	80%
At-home recovery				✓			✓		✓	✓
Prescription drugs								Basic	Basic	Extended
Preventive screening					✓					✓

Source: Guide to Health Insurance for People With Medicare, published by the U.S. Department of Health and Human Services.

who has certified the home health care plan. You should discuss the various benefit requirements and limitations with your physician. Currently, the at-home recovery benefit pays a maximum $40 per visit for up to seven visits per week and can be used up to eight weeks after Medicare's home health care visits stop. The maximum benefit is $1,600 per calendar year.

- Prescription drugs. It pays 50 percent of the cost, up to a maximum $1,250 annually, after the policyholder meets a $250 annual deductible.
- Extended prescription drug coverage. It pays 50 percent of the cost of outpatient prescription drugs, up to a maximum annual benefit of $3,000 after the policyholder meets a $250 annual deductible.
- Preventive screening. This benefit pays up to $120 per year for physician-ordered health care screenings, such as diabetes screenings and thyroid function tests.

Q. Do I need to buy a Medigap policy?

A. Medicare beneficiaries enrolled in managed-care plans (HMOs) or who are eligible for Medicaid usually do not need Medigap insurance. Also, if you have insurance from an employer or a labor union, you probably won't need it.

Q. Can I get a Medigap policy even if I have a medical condition?

A. Yes. CMS regulations mandate that when you first enroll in Medicare Part B, you have six months to select a Medigap policy. During that time, you cannot be rejected for health reasons. The insurer can exclude coverage for a pre-existing condition, however, for up to six months.

Q. Among Medigap policies, which ones make the most sense?

A. For basic coverage, "A" is by far the least expensive and provides protection against disastrous expenses. But some professionals recommend more extensive—and more expensive—coverage. Policy F, which is the most popular choice, may cost over twice as much as an "A" policy because "F" offers coverage for skilled nursing co-payments, health emergencies in foreign countries and excess doctors' charges. Policy "I" offers these benefits as well as prescription drug coverage, so it might be a good buy for people who expect to pay $700 or more per year for drugs.

Q. Can I buy any of the 10 standardized packages?

A. Not necessarily. Insurers must make Plan A available if they sell any of the other plans in a particular state; however, they are not required to offer all the plans approved for sale by any given state. Thus far, most insurance companies have opted to sell only a few and are reluctant to offer some of the more comprehensive plans because of the potential cost. They believe that only the very ill would be likely to pay the extremely high premiums they would have to charge for such comprehensive coverage. Furthermore, even high premiums wouldn't guarantee the insurer a break-even point, let alone a profit.

Additionally, some states, such as Massachusetts, Minnesota and Wisconsin, were granted waivers from the regulations because they already had their own standardization programs for Medigap insurance. Thus, consumers in those states can choose from standardized policies, but the benefit packages are different from those in the 10 standard plans. If you live in one of these states, contact your state insurance department to find out what supplemental coverage is available.

Q. If I bought a Medigap policy before the policies were standardized in 1992, will I have to switch to one of the new standard policies?

A. That's up to your state. If you have an older policy that is guaranteed renewable, the federal requirements don't apply to it. But some states have adopted regulations that affect existing nonstandard policies. For example, some require or permit insurers to convert older policies to one of the new standardized plans. Check with your state insurance department to find out the requirements.

➤ **Observation:** Some older policies provide superior coverage, especially for prescription drugs and extended skilled nursing care. Before you switch, compare the benefits and premiums. Also, check to see if there are waiting periods for any of the benefits in the new policy. If you've had your old policy for at least six months, the new policy may not impose a waiting period for a pre-existing condition if you satisfied the waiting period for a similar benefit under your old policy. But it may impose a waiting period of up to six months for benefits that were not in your old policy.

Q. What if I switch and then decide I prefer my old policy?

A. If you switch, you won't be permitted to return to a nonstandard policy. Be sure to compare coverage before you switch policies.

Q. What will I have to pay for a Medigap policy?

A. That will depend on your age and the benefits you want. Expect to pay at least $350 annually for a limited policy, while a comprehensive policy can approach $10,000 a year. You should shop carefully, too. In Florida a basic "A" policy might cost under $800 per year or more than $2,600 per year, depending on the company.

What explains such huge differentials? One reason may lie in marketing strategy. If an insurer wants to focus on policy "A," it may quote higher premiums for its other policies and be very competitive when it comes to "A." In addition, some insurers may charge higher premiums based on their company's financial strength, say, or based on the consumer's ability to switch among policies without having to take a medical exam.

Perhaps more important is the way in which policies are priced. Some companies use an "issue age" approach, meaning that you pay a level premium that's determined by your age when you bought the policy. If the company wants to raise your premium, it has to raise the premiums of everyone else holding similar policies.

Other companies use an "attained age" method, with relatively low initial premiums that increase as policyholders grow older. Still others charge the same rates for everyone, regardless of age—a system that benefits older consumers at the expense of younger ones.

Thus, you should check to see if your premiums are scheduled to increase as you grow older; that's the case with many seemingly inexpensive policies.

Note: The same financial and demographic pressures that were behind the push for Medicare reform are being felt by companies that offer Medigap policies. As a result, premiums have been rising rapidly.

Q. If I find a good Medigap policy, am I still responsible for paying some of the costs?

A. Yes. Certain kinds of care, charges and supplies are not covered by Medicare or most Medigap policies. Among these are private-duty nursing, costs associated with skilled nursing home care beyond 100 days a year, part-time nursing home care and custodial care in a nursing home or at home. Also exempt are routine physical exams, routine foot care, eye exams, most immunizations, cosmetic surgery, chiropractic treatments and dental care.

The most burdensome charges are usually doctor bills above Medicare's approved amount. Only a few Medigap policies cover these. To avoid these potentially high charges, ask doctors or medical suppliers, such as laboratories and therapists, if they participate in Medicare or accept assignment of Medicare benefits: that is, accept the Medicare payment as full payment for their services. (Participating doctors accept assignment on all Medicare claims.)

Q. Should I buy a Medigap policy or join a Medicare HMO?

A. The Medigap/traditional Medicare combination might be a better deal than a Medicare HMO, at least for those who can afford Medigap policies. If you have a strong relationship with a primary care physician, you may not want to enroll in an HMO that is not affiliated with your physician. Also, specialist referrals may be difficult to obtain, and HMOs may not be good choices for retirees who travel extensively.

By contrast, people who have been in HMOs before retirement may find it easy to adjust to a Medicare HMO. Retirees who relocate won't be familiar with doctors in their new locale, so they might prefer a Medicare HMO. In addition, Medicare HMOs cost less and don't involve much paperwork.

Some experts recommend keeping a Medigap policy for a while after joining a Medicare HMO to make sure you are happy with the new plan. This may help you avoid higher premiums, waiting periods or even denial by a Medigap insurer if you want to return to regular Medicare.

Q. Do military retirees need Medigap policies?

A. Not necessarily. In 2001, the federal government announced "the most sweeping improvements to the Department of Defense's health care system in nearly 30 years" under a plan called TRICARE For Life. If you are a uniformed services beneficiary (a retiree or a family member) who has attained the age of 65, are Medicare eligible and have purchased Medicare Part B, TRICARE For Life provides a permanent health care benefit. As a result, some eligible parties are canceling their Medigap policies in favor of this free coverage.

Q. How did the 1997 Balanced Budget Act affect Medigap policies?

A. If you lose your Medigap coverage, either through events beyond your control (the company dropped out of the business, for example) or because you moved away from the coverage area, you will have 63 days to buy a new "A," "B," "C" or "F" policy, regardless of your health. Lower-cost, high-deductible versions of "F" and "J" have been approved as well; their availability depends on action by individual states.

Q. What if I discover that the policy I bought duplicates coverage I already have?

A. From 1990 until late 1994, you didn't have to worry about that. Insurance consumer legislation enacted in 1990 allowed federal criminal and civil penalties to be imposed against any company or agent that knowingly sold a policy duplicating the coverage you already had under Medicare or a Medigap policy. But in 1994 Congress passed regulations once again allowing insurers to sell policies that duplicate Medicare or Medigap coverage as long as they disclose this fact. This means that Medicare participants have to read the fine print to make sure they are not buying a policy that duplicates coverage.

➤ **Recommendation:** Take advantage of the free-look provision: Insurance companies must give you at least 30 days to review a Medigap policy. If you decide you don't want it, return it to the agent or company within 30 days and ask for a full refund of the premiums you paid. If you have any trouble getting your money back, contact your state insurance regulator *(see listings in Appendix II)*.

Q. How do I locate Medigap insurers?

A. To find out which companies offer Medigap policies in your state, call your local Social Security office or go online to ***www.medicare.gov*** and click on "Medical Personal Plan Finder." If you'd like advice on which Medigap policy is best for you, call your state's insurance department or agency on aging and request information about its insurance counseling program.

Beware of Medigap sales pitches

State and federal laws govern the sale of Medigap insurance. Penalties may be imposed against any insurance company or agent that knowingly engages in the following activities:

- Tells you that they are employees or agents of the Medicare program or of any government agency.
- Makes a false statement that a policy meets legal standards for certification when it does not.
- Sells you a Medigap policy that is not one of the approved standard policies.
- Uses the U.S. mail for advertising or delivering health insurance policies to supplement Medicare if the policies have not been approved for sale in that state.
- Denies you open enrollment when you are entitled to it.

Caution: Your doctor might offer you a "retainer agreement" under which he will provide certain non-Medicare-covered services and waive the Medicare co-insurance and deductible amounts. This arrangement may violate the federal laws governing Medigap policies. If a doctor refuses to see you as a Medicare patient unless you pay him an annual fee and sign a retainer agreement, you should report this potentially illegal activity to your state insurance department.

For more information on Medigap, contact your state insurance department or Social Security office and request the *Guide to Health Insurance for People With Medicare* (also available online at ***www.medicare.gov/Publications/Home.asp***).

Fraud Hotline

If you believe that you have been the victim of illegal sales practices by insurance companies, you should contact your state insurance department or federal authorities. The Inspector General at the U.S. Department of Health and Human Services maintains a fraud hotline at (800) 447-8477.

If you suspect that a health care provider may be billing Medicare for services you did not receive, you should contact your Medicare carrier or fiscal intermediary (listed at the top of your Medicare Summary Notice). You may get a reward of $1,000 for reporting Medicare fraud and abuse if your report leads directly to the recovery of at least $100 by Medicare.

5

Medicare Advantage Replaces Medicare+Choice

With great fanfare, the government unveiled the Medicare+ Choice program in 1997. Besides traditional fee-for-service Medicare, beneficiaries were to be given a number of private health plan choices, ranging from HMOs, provider-sponsored organizations (PSOs) and preferred provider organizations (PPOs) to medical savings accounts (MSAs) and private fee-for-service plans.

Some of these choices, though, have hardly left the drawing board. As of January 2004, there were no Medicare MSAs in place and only a smattering of PSOs and private fee-for-service plans, with relatively few Medicare beneficiaries. Also, some PPO demonstration projects are under way.

Under the 2003 Medicare law, an expanded program, Medicare Advantage, has replaced Medicare+Choice. The new program, making extensive use of PPOs, eventually will be modeled on the health insurance system provided for members of Congress as well as millions of federal employees and retirees. The Federal Employees Health Benefits Program invites health plans to submit a package of benefits at a proposed cost and then negotiates prices and benefits with each plan. If approved, the plan then goes on the menu offered to federal workers and retirees.

Such a system may be incorporated into Medicare Advantage in the future. For now, though, Medicare Advantage consists mainly of two alternatives: traditional Medicare and HMOs.

Some HMOs Are Retreating

The 1997 Balanced Budget Act restricted payments to Medicare HMOs in an effort to strengthen Medicare's finances. At the same time, regulations and compliance procedures were tightened. In response, some managed-care plans announced that they would cut back their Medicare participation.

On Jan. 1, 2004, about 41,000 people were dropped by HMOs that pulled out of Medicare (those were in addition to the 2.3 million who had already been dropped since 1998). Altogether, 16 plans either withdrew from Medicare or reduced their service areas.

Beneficiaries who are dropped by a Medicare HMO can enroll in another—if they can find one. Of the 41,000 people recently dropped by Medicare+Choice plans, 3,000 don't have another one in their area, but half of them will be eligible to enroll in one of the PPO demonstration projects. Currently, some states lack any Medicare Advantage plans while several others have only a private fee-for-service plan rather than any Medicare HMOs.

Medical Savings Accounts for Seniors

Since 1997 medical savings accounts have been available in the private sector to workers in small companies and to the self-employed. These "medical IRAs" are tax-advantaged accounts typically used in conjunction with catastrophic (high-deductible) health insurance. MSAs are intended to discourage people from over-utilizing medical insurance benefits by having individuals assume some financial risk in return for the tax savings.

Medicare MSAs were first scheduled to be offered as a test program, limited to 390,000 Medicare beneficiaries. But the 2003 Medicare law has made MSAs a permanent option for seniors, with no deadline for signing up and no restrictions on total enrollment.

Thus, Medicare beneficiaries will have the MSA as an option if a private company offers such a plan. (As of January 2004, no company had applied to provide Medicare MSAs.)

In theory, here's how a Medicare MSA would work:

You would select a Medicare MSA health insurance policy, which has a high deductible, and set up an MSA account at a bank or other financial institution. Medicare would pay the premium to the insurance plan and make a deposit into your MSA. So you would have tax-free cash in your MSA, which could be invested with a bank, broker, mutual fund and so forth. Buildup inside the MSA would be tax free, as would withdrawals to pay your medical expenses. (Nonmedical withdrawals would be subject to tax.) Any surplus in your account would be added to the following year's deposit from Medicare. Once the deductible was satisfied, your insurance coverage would pay for additional medical care. (You would still be responsible for paying Medicare's monthly Part B premium.)

Depending on which MSA insurance plan you chose, you might be limited to a network of doctors, or you might be able to go to any doctor or hospital. You might be asked to pay extra charges by doctors, hospitals and other providers who don't accept the insurer's fee as payment in full.

Medicare MSAs may appeal to people in good health who like the idea of building up their account for future use. You may have some financial exposure, though, if the money in the MSA isn't enough to cover your medical bills.

Health Savings Accounts for Workers Under 65

The new Medicare law also creates Health Savings Accounts for people not yet covered by Medicare. Effective in 2004, workers under age 65 who have high-deductible health insurance policies can make tax-deductible contributions to their own HSA. They'll be able to make tax-free withdrawals to pay medical bills while money not withdrawn can accumulate tax free until needed.

If the HSA is set up as an employer-sponsored plan, employer contributions will be made on a pre-tax basis and won't be taxable to the employee. Unlike flexible spending accounts, HSAs will be portable if you change jobs and the assets may be rolled over, year after year. Thus you could draw on them to cover not only current health costs but also medical care during retirement.

Note: If the new HSAs become popular, they might lead insurers to offer MSAs to Medicare participants. *(See box, page 54.)*

Even if you can find a Medicare HMO to join, expect to face restrictions on prescription drug coverage. In some states, no Medicare HMOs offer a prescription benefit while some other states have only one plan, in one county, that covers drugs. Moreover, even the Medicare HMOs that offer drug coverage are charging co-payments for prescriptions and placing dollar caps on the coverage.

At the same time, Medicare HMOs are eliminating (or charging much more for) coverage for eyeglasses and dental care while sharply raising premiums. In 2003, the Commonwealth Fund estimated that the average out-of-pocket cost for Medicare HMO enrollees was $1,964, compared to $976 in 1999. HMOs contend these changes are necessary because of rising costs and inadequate reimbursements.

The 2003 Medicare law contains $12 billion to entice private insurers to join or remain in the Medicare Advantage program. The Bush administration has indicated that it wants private insurers to play a larger role in Medicare. Higher reimbursements may help Medicare Advantage resume its growth.

In 1997, about 18 percent of Medicare beneficiaries had enrolled in Medicare+Choice plans. (At that time, the government projected enrollment would almost double by 2002.) To control costs, Congress changed the Medicare+Choice payment formula, but the new formula hasn't worked: Beneficiary enrollment has dropped to 11 percent of all Medicare participants. Since 2000, more than 2 million beneficiaries have lost their Medicare+Choice coverage as plans dropped out of the program, while other enrollees are seeing their benefits shrink.

Medicare has taken steps to ensure that beneficiaries affected by retreating HMOs will have options. Insurers must guarantee access to certain Medigap plans for beneficiaries who are being forced to change their health care coverage, regardless of their prior use of health care services or their current medical conditions. Also, to make the transition easier for these beneficiaries, the plans leaving Medicare must provide clear information on other health care options.

Keep in mind that people leaving Medicare HMOs can always enroll in the traditional fee-for-service Medicare plan. However, until 2006, Medicare won't cover prescription drugs. By contrast, 70 percent of those enrolled in Medicare HMOs receive some prescription drug benefit. Meanwhile, those enrolled in traditional Medicare may buy Medigap policies with a drug benefit, but such policies are expensive (they can cost nearly $10,000 per year) and acceptance is not guaranteed. Or, they can purchase drug discount cards until the drug benefit plan kicks in under Medicare.

To help seniors compare managed-care plans, CMS publishes the booklet *Medicare & You*. For further assistance in evaluating Medicare HMOs, you can call (800) MEDICARE and ask them to send you information on quality and member satisfaction. Or visit ***www.medicare.gov*** and click on "Medical Personal Plan Finder." You can also contact any Medicare HMO and ask for statistics about grievances and appeals that have been filed.

6

Long-Term-Care Policies

It's hard to predict whether you will ever need nursing home care. But as several studies indicate, about 40 percent of Americans will be in a nursing home at some point. The average stay in a nursing home lasts about two and a half years, but there's a 10 percent risk that a person will stay more than four years. Yet, despite the fear of needing long-term care, less than 10 percent of Americans' nursing home bills are paid by private long-term-care (LTC) policies.

Medicaid pays about 50 percent of nursing home bills, Medicare covers 10 percent (for skilled nursing care), and individuals pay the balance out of pocket. The "cognitively impaired" elderly—about a fourth of the Medicare population—need supervision and custodial care (assistance with daily living tasks), which Medicare won't cover. Because women tend to outnumber men in nursing homes, they are more likely to need custodial care.

Long-term-care policies have become more popular since a 1996 law afforded them tax treatment similar to that of health insurance policies. Benefits received under such policies, up to $230 per day (in 2004), won't be considered taxable income. In addition, premiums paid for LTC policies can be counted as medical expenses by those who itemize deductions on their tax returns. In 2004 people over age 70 can include as much as $3,250 worth of LTC premiums as deductible medical outlays; the limits scale down by age, reaching $260 for those 40 or younger. (These limits will rise each year to keep pace with inflation.) If your total medical expenses (including LTC premiums up to the age-appropriate limits) exceed 7.5 percent of your AGI, your LTC premiums will be deductible expenses.

A Complicated Decision

Deciding whether to buy a long-term-care policy can be complicated. Premiums generally are lower for those who are in better health and younger than age 60. For those with high incomes and substantial assets, the answer may be different from that of people with lower incomes and fewer assets. Strategies also differ for those who are single versus married, in their 60s and in good health or in their 80s with chronic ailments. Generally, LTC policies are best for people with middle incomes. It is unlikely that lower-income people can afford the cost of such insurance, and the very wealthy have incomes that can cover the annual costs of nursing home care.

A general rule-of-thumb is that your premiums for an LTC policy should not exceed 6 percent of your income. Additionally, it is usually not worth the money to buy coverage for more than three years of long-term care because the average stay in a nursing home is less than three years.

Your best bet is to consult a financial adviser, who can help you determine the strategy that fits your needs. At one time, few financial advisers considered such insurance a good investment; instead, they usually recommended investing some of your assets at higher rates of return to increase your total net worth. That strategy creates a cushion, in case you suddenly face mammoth medical bills. But today's better policies—with fewer restrictions and coverage that allows expanded care—have prompted some financial advisers to take a second look at the benefits of LTC policies. Moreover, full medical coverage delivers peace of mind—particularly for those who dislike uncertainty—about a problem that most of us, understandably, find upsetting to contemplate.

To buy complete coverage, you should elect both Part A (hospital) and Part B (medical) Medicare coverage, and buy both a supplemental Medigap policy and a long-term-care policy.

You should plan, however, to review these policies at least once a year to ensure that your benefits keep pace with inflation and to compare them with any new insurance policies that might be better tailored to your needs. New insurance products are often less expensive and more comprehensive than older ones, but be aware that if you change policies, you may trigger new waiting periods for pre-existing conditions.

The Basics of LTC Policies

Many issues are involved in buying LTC policies. The following questions address the major ones.

Q. Now that I have Medicare and a Medigap policy, am I fully covered for nursing home care?

A. No. The combination of Medicare and Medigap policies pays for only a limited amount of skilled nursing care. That's the kind of daily nursing and rehabilitative care that follows a hospital stay and is the direct result of a doctor's orders. Medicare will also pay for short-term, intermittent skilled care at home if various—and increasingly strict—conditions are met and a doctor sets up the home health care regimen for you.

But you will not be covered if you need intermediate or custodial nursing home care or prolonged health care in your home. "Intermediate care" is defined as skilled care that isn't required on a daily basis but is performed by medical personnel under a doctor's orders. "Custodial care" is defined as help with the activities of daily living (ADLs), such as bathing, dressing and eating. "Prolonged home health care" also assists with ADLs and may include the part-time services of aides or help from homemakers or chore workers.

Q. What can I expect to pay for such care?

A. The cost is astonishing. On average, staying in a nursing home costs more than $180 per day, and in some areas $80,000 a year is the norm. The bill in some areas of the United States can balloon to more than $100,000 annually. Moreover, the large majority of nursing home patients need custodial care, not skilled care, which means Medicare won't contribute a penny. Multiply the average monthly cost ($5,400) by the average length of stay (30 months) and you could be out of pocket $162,000. Even hiring unskilled aides to assist you at home three times a week with simple chores, such as dressing and grooming, can easily cost you $600 a month, or $7,200 a year.

Q. Could nursing home care eat up my entire estate?

A. Yes, if you don't plan for this contingency. This is a difficult and emotional issue for older Americans. You've worked hard all your life to build a nest egg or to establish an estate to pass along to your heirs. A lengthy stay in a nursing home could consume all your assets. What's more, most elderly parents want to avoid being a financial burden to their grown children.

An estate planner, especially the lawyer who drew up your will or trusts, can advise you on how to handle this situation. There may be some financial strategies your lawyer can employ that will preserve some of your estate and still provide for your care if you should find yourself without adequate protection.

Q. What protection is available if I should need nursing home or home care services?

A. More than 120 health insurance companies, including a number of Blue Cross/Blue Shield plans, sell LTC insurance. Most of the policies are indemnity policies paying a fixed amount per day for care in a nursing home or for home health care. The home health benefit might be one-half the nursing home benefit: $40–$75 per day, for example, versus a nursing home benefit of $80–$150 per day.

Home health care programs may include adult day care, respite care (short-term care in a rest home or nursing home to give caretakers at home a break), aide or chore services and companion visits. If you are considering this kind of policy, take care not to duplicate the coverage of a skilled nursing facility provided by Medicare, Medigap or a prepayment plan.

Average LTC Insurance Costs

The costs of long-term-care policies depend on your age, your health and the deductibles and benefits you choose. Following are some averages provided by the Health Insurance Association of America in Washington, D.C.

These rates apply to policies from the top 11 LTC sellers, which account for most of the LTC policies sold. The policies offer daily benefits of $100, a 20-day elimination period and four years of coverage. Most pay for skilled and intermediate nursing, as well as custodial care.

	Average Annual Premium	
Buyer's Age	**Base Plan***	**With Inflation Protection****
40	$ 310	$ 641
50	401	849
65	996	1,726
79	4,180	5,821

*Without inflation protection.
**With lifetime 5 percent per year compound inflation protection.
Source: Health Insurance Association of America.

Q. Will an LTC policy cover all my expenses?

A. No policy provides blanket coverage for all expenses, and most are not automatically adjusted for inflation. This means that benefits will lag behind increases in medical costs. To guard against having your benefits eroded by inflation, consider buying a policy with an option for inflation protection. Also, you will want to review your policy annually, compare it with other policies on the market and switch if it makes sense.

Caution: Take a close look at the new policy's exclusions and waiting period for coverage of pre-existing conditions. When you switch LTC policies, you start the clock ticking all over again. So if you should have to go into a nursing home during the waiting period because of a pre-existing condition, the policy will not pay benefits.

Q. Would I have to be hospitalized before an LTC policy would pay for custodial nursing care?

A. Policies differ. Many of those issued before 1990 stipulated that a policyholder had to be hospitalized first to receive benefits for a nursing home. Others demanded that you receive skilled or intermediate care before they would pay for custodial expenses. Newer policies do not contain such stipulations on eligibility. Because most custodial-care patients do not require prior hospitalization or skilled nursing care, be sure to shop for a policy free of these restrictions.

Standards for LTC Policies

The National Association of Insurance Commissioners has developed standards for LTC policies, which include the following:

At least one year of nursing home or home health care coverage, including intermediate and custodial care.

Coverage for Alzheimer's disease if the policyholder should develop the condition after purchasing the policy.

An option for inflation protection, with a choice among the following: automatic annual increase in initial benefit level, such as 5 percent a year; a guaranteed right to increase benefit levels periodically without providing evidence of insurability; and coverage of a specific percentage of actual or reasonable charges.

No stipulations for prior levels of care to collect benefits.

A guarantee that the policy cannot be canceled, nonrenewed or otherwise terminated because you get older or suffer a deterioration in physical or mental health.

An outline of coverage that systematically describes the policy's benefits, limitations and exclusions—thereby allowing you to compare it with other policies on a uniform basis.

An LTC insurance shopper's guide to help you decide whether LTC coverage is appropriate for you.

The right to return the policy within 30 days after purchase for any reason and receive a full premium refund.

➤ **Observation:** Most LTC policies require that any facility you choose be licensed by the state and participate in Medicaid and Medicare.

Q. What other factors should I look at in evaluating nursing home insurance policies?

A. Among the most important factors are the following:

✔ **Breadth of coverage.** There are no "standard" benefits, so it is difficult to compare policies offered by different companies. Some policies limit coverage to services provided in nursing homes, while others cover both nursing home and home health care. It is probably best to have a policy that covers skilled, intermediate and custodial nursing home care, along with custodial care in the patient's home. It also should cover Alzheimer's disease and other organic, cognitive disabilities.

➤ **Observation:** Because of the potential for fraud and the difficulty of monitoring benefits, many insurance companies will not pay benefits when family members perform home care services. However, some policies, including group policies sold to employers, do offer some coverage allowing family members to provide care.

- ✔ **Duration of benefits.** LTC policies typically limit benefits to a maximum dollar amount or a maximum number of days. Separate benefit limits are usually set for nursing homes and home health care. Typical benefit periods for nursing homes are two, three, four or five years or for life. If payments aren't for life, check whether the policy provides for continuation of benefits (provides that any unused portion of the daily benefit will remain in a pool to extend the policy's benefit period) or an alternate plan of care (allows the policyholder to use the nursing home benefit to pay for home health care).

Insurers define maximum benefit periods in two ways. Under one, the policy offers a one-time maximum benefit period, such as five years. When that total is reached—either in one long stay or several shorter stays—the benefits cease. Under the other definition, a policy would cover multiple stays of up to five years each, provided that the stays are separated by six months or more. Under home care provisions, the benefit period is usually more limited than for nursing home stays, and benefit periods of one to two years are available.

- ✔ **Waiver of payments.** Look for a policy stipulating that you won't have to pay premiums while you are receiving benefits. Some companies stop billing you as they make the benefit payment. Others wait 60 to 90 days. Often, premiums are not waived while you are in a hospital or if you are receiving care at home.
- ✔ **Renewability.** Most individual LTC policies are guaranteed renewable, although the premium can be increased if it is raised for an entire group of policyholders. As long as you disclose all the information required on your original application and pay your premiums on time, your policy can't be canceled, even if your health worsens after you buy the policy. Don't buy a policy that lacks this protection.
- ✔ **Limitations and exclusions.** All policies have limitations and exclusions. You should carefully scrutinize those based on age, deductible (or elimination) periods before the policy begins paying benefits (during which the policyholder bears the full cost), and the amount and duration of benefits. Others to consider include pre-existing conditions. Most policies refuse to pay benefits for an ailment or injury that already exists, or for one that occurs in the first six months after the policy has been issued.
- ✔ **Eligibility.** After a certain age, you will be unable to buy a policy. The limit is usually about 84, although some policies are available through age 99 if your health is good.
- ✔ **Specific exclusions.** Policies may not pay for long-term care related to mental or nervous conditions, alcoholism, drug abuse, mental retardation, certain other health conditions and self-inflicted injuries.
- ✔ **Prior levels of care.** As mentioned earlier, some policies will pay for whatever level of care you need. Others require a certain period of nursing home

care before you are eligible for home care, or skilled care before you are eligible for custodial nursing home care. Look for a policy with no prior-care stipulations.

➤ **Recommendation:** Read and compare policies carefully before you buy. Don't rely on what you read in the sales literature. Also, check each insurer's financial stability. Do business only with companies that have "A+" or "A" financial ratings. Several private companies or rating agencies conduct financial analyses of insurance companies and grade them. These ratings carry no guarantee of accuracy regarding a company's future stability, but they can provide information on how some analysts view the health of particular insurance companies. Agencies use various rating scales, so be sure to find out how the agency labels its highest rating. Ratings from some agencies are available at most public libraries, or you can contact the agencies listed below:

Demotech, Inc.
(614) 761-8602; ***www.demotech.com***

Fitch, Inc.
(212) 908-0500; ***www.fitchratings.com***

Moody's Investors Service
(212) 553-1653; ***www.moodys.com***

Standard & Poor's
(212) 438-2000; ***www.standardandpoors.com***

Weiss Research, Inc.
(800) 289-9222; ***www.weissratings.com***

A.M. Best Company
(908) 439-2200; ***www.ambest.com***

A special report, *Insurance Ratings: Comparison of Private Agency Ratings for Life/Health Insurers*, is issued by the General Accounting Office. You may find it worthwhile to order this free report (GAO/GGD-94-204BR) by writing to the GAO, P.O. Box 37050, Washington, DC 20013 or calling (202) 512-3000.

Q. Is there anything else I need to consider?

A. Before buying LTC insurance, take an inventory of the costs of long-term care in your area and the resources you could apply to your LTC needs. For example, do you have savings, life insurance or a pension that would help pay your costs? Would or could other family members help if necessary? Do you qualify for community services? Remember, also, that if the premiums are too costly for your income, you probably are better off forgoing LTC insurance. If you did face the possibility of nursing home care, you would have to use up your savings, but then you would qualify for Medicaid, which would pay for your care.

Q. Should I wait until I am near retirement to shop for a policy?

A. No. You will save money by buying when you're younger. For example, a 50-year-old who bought an $80-per-day policy with inflation protection of 5 percent compounded for $802 a year would pay about $20,000 in premiums over a 25-year average life expectancy. A 65-year-old would pay nearly $27,500 for the same policy over his 15-year life expectancy. Another possible disadvantage of waiting until you're older to obtain coverage is that you risk incurring a condition (such as Parkinson's disease) that would make it virtually impossible for you to buy a policy.

Q. How else can I save money on an LTC policy?

A. Opt for a longer deductible period before your benefits begin (90 days, for example, instead of 20). Elect a shorter payout (three years, for example, instead of five). Forgo coverage for home care if your resources are sufficient to pay for home care without insurance benefits. You could also save between 25 percent and 60 percent by eliminating inflation protection; but considering the escalating costs of health care, this option might well leave you with insufficient coverage.

There's still another possibility if you have an ongoing need for life insurance. Buy a life insurance policy with an LTC rider in lieu of an LTC policy. Under a life insurance policy's living benefits or accelerated provisions, the policy will pay benefits if the policyholder is confined to a nursing home. Benefits paid during the policyholder's lifetime are deducted from the death benefit.

Shopping for Medical Insurance in General

Obviously, the more protection you want, the more you will pay for a policy. You must weigh cost versus benefit. Here are some guidelines to follow:

- **Shop carefully before you buy.** Policies differ widely in coverage and cost. If you have determined that you would benefit from a health care policy—whether Medigap, LTC or another plan—contact several companies and compare their policies. Be sure to compare benefits, types of facilities you have to be in to receive coverage, coverage limitations, exclusions and, of course, the premiums. *Note:* Policies that provide identical coverage and benefits may not necessarily cost the same.
- **Don't buy more policies than you need.** Duplicate coverage is costly and unnecessary. A single, comprehensive policy is better than several with overlapping coverage.
- **Consider your alternatives.** To meet your health care needs better, consider (1) continuing the group coverage you have at work; (2) joining a managed-care plan; (3) buying a Medigap policy; or (4) buying a long-term-care policy.
- **Check for exclusions of pre-existing conditions.** Many policies exclude coverage for pre-existing health problems. These are generally defined as conditions for which medical advice was given or treatment received within six months before the effective date of your coverage. Don't be misled by the phrase "no medical examination required." It doesn't exempt you from the rule. In fact, your policy can be canceled if the insurer discovers that you failed to disclose a pre-existing condition when you applied for your policy. State laws require Medigap policies to pick up the cost for pre-existing conditions after the policy

has been in effect for six months, but you could be at considerable financial risk during those six months. Look for a policy that waives the exclusion or has a shorter waiting period.

- **Be cautious about replacing existing coverage.** Be suspicious of any suggestion that you give up your policy and buy a replacement. Often the new policy will impose waiting periods or will have exclusions. Nonetheless, don't hold onto inadequate policies simply because you have had them a long time. Only switch for different benefits, better service or a better price.
- **Be aware of maximum benefits.** Most policies set some limit on benefits, either in dollars or in the number of days for which payment will be made. Keep in mind that some insurance policies (but not Medigap policies) pay nothing or less than the Medicare-approved amount for hospital outpatient medical services or services in a doctor's office.
- **Check your right to renew.** Beware of policies that allow a company to refuse renewal of your policy—these provide the least permanent coverage. Look for a policy that can be renewed automatically.
- **Make sure you know what you're buying.** Be aware that policies to supplement Medicare are not sold or serviced by the federal or state governments. State insurance departments approve policies sold by insurance companies, but approval means only that the company and policy meet the requirements of state law. For example, do not believe statements claiming that insurance to supplement Medicare is a government-sponsored program. If anyone tells you that she is from the government and later tries to sell you an insurance policy, report that person to your state insurance department or to federal authorities. This claim violates federal and state laws.

Quality Indicators: Nursing Home Care

The government publishes data on the quality of care in nursing homes to spur improvements and provide consumers with information about their long-term health care options. You can get quality indicators on U.S. nursing homes by going to ***www.medicare.gov*** and clicking on "Nursing Home Compare."

CMS uses 10 quality measures: six for long-term nursing home residents and four for short-stay residents. For long-term residents, who stay in a nursing home an average of two to three years, the data show the percentage with pain, infections and in physical restraints. For short-term patients, whose stays average three to four weeks, the data show how many maintain or improve their ability to walk while in a nursing home, as well as the percentage with delirium and pain.

Information is available also on staffing levels as well as on deficiencies found during annual inspections and complaint investigations.

Over the past few years, the Medicare Web site has been beefed up, standardized and made easier to use. Thus, families need not rely solely on hospital discharge planners to help them decide where to take an elderly relative who can no longer live on his own. The Web site will give you an idea of what's available in your area. This information may be especially helpful in identifying homes where care is inadequate.

■ **Know whom you're dealing with.** A company must meet certain qualifications to do business. Agents have to be licensed by your state and should carry identification showing their name and company. If an agent cannot verify that he is licensed, take your business elsewhere. A business card is not a license.

■ **Take your time.** Don't let a short enrollment period pressure you. (Professional salespeople will not rush you.) Allow yourself time to think through your decision. If you question whether a program is worthwhile, ask the salesperson to explain it to a friend or a relative whose judgment you respect.

■ **Look for an outline of coverage.** You must be given a clearly worded summary of any policy you are considering. Read it carefully and use it for comparison shopping.

■ **Do not pay cash.** Pay by check, money order or bank draft made payable to the insurance company, not to the agent. Get a receipt with the company's name, address and phone number.

Further Information

You may want to send for the free booklet, *Guide to Health Insurance for People With Medicare*. It is available from CMS at (800) 633-4227; request Publication 02110. Keep in mind that if you are shopping for a Medigap policy, the Medigap insurance carriers are required to provide this publication. CMS also provides a booklet titled *Guide to Choosing a Nursing Home* (Publication 02174).

Medicare's Web site (***www.medicare.gov***) also carries up-to-date information on these topics:

- **"Nursing Home Compare."** You can get information on the 17,000 nursing homes participating in Medicare and Medicaid, including the number and type of residents, facility ownership, staffing levels and mix, and each facility's rating compared to state and national averages.
- **"Prescription Drug Assistance Programs."** You'll find information on how to apply for drug assistance provided by pharmaceutical companies, states, community-based programs and disease-specific programs. It also allows you to search by your ZIP Code for drug coverage benefits offered by supplemental Medigap plans and Medicare managed-care plans in your community.
- **"Participating Physician Directory."** This directory will help you find doctors who see Medicare patients. You can search by specialty and location among the 90 percent of all U.S. physicians who, as participating providers, accept Medicare payment rates and charge beneficiaries only the standard 20 percent co-insurance rate.

Also, the National Association of Insurance Commissioners (NAIC) publishes *A Shopper's Guide to Long-Term Care Insurance*. To order, phone (816) 783-8300 or visit the NAIC Web site at ***www.naic.org***.

7

Your Rights as a Medicare Patient

Just because you have Medicare doesn't mean you have lost your rights as a patient. In fact, at the end of this section we present a sample notice that all hospitals are required to provide to Medicare patients. The following questions and answers focus on your rights under Medicare.

Q. Can I be forced out of the hospital by Medicare before I feel ready to leave?

A. Yes. When you are admitted to a Medicare-participating hospital, you will receive a document entitled "An Important Message From Medicare" *(see end of this section)*. This brochure explains your rights as a hospital patient and provides the name, address and phone number of the peer review organization (PRO) for your state. It is up to the PRO to decide whether you need hospital treatment and whether the treatment you are getting is appropriate and of good quality.

Q. What if I disagree with the PRO's decision?

A. If you feel that you have been improperly refused admission to a hospital or that you have been forced to leave too soon, ask for a written explanation of the decision. Medicare regulations require that a written notice:

- Explain fully how you can appeal the decision.
- Provide you with the name, address and phone number of the PRO where you can submit your appeal or request for review.

If you disagree with the PRO's initial decision, you can appeal by requesting a reconsideration. If you disagree with the PRO's reconsideration and the amount in question is $200 or more, you can request a hearing by an administrative law judge. Cases involving $2,000 or more can eventually be appealed to a federal court.

If you belong to an HMO, it will usually make the decisions about your hospital care. In most cases, you do not have the right to appeal the HMO's decision to a PRO. You do have the right, however, to register complaints about the quality of your hospital to your state's PRO, and you can request a reconsideration from your HMO. If your HMO does not rule in your favor, it must forward your request for reconsideration to CMS for a review and determination.

Federal law requires Medicare-certified HMOs to provide a written explanation of appeal rights at the time of enrollment and at least once a year thereafter. If you have not received a written explanation, you should request one from your plan's membership office. Or write to CMS, 7500 Security Blvd., Baltimore, MD 21244-1850 or visit *www.cms.gov*.

Q. Can I be refused Medicare coverage for care provided at skilled nursing homes, home health care services and hospices?

A. Yes. When a provider believes that Medicare will not pay for its services, it will send you a written notice explaining why. This notice is not an official Medicare determination. If you want one, you can ask the provider to file a claim on your behalf with Medicare (the provider is required by law to do so). You will receive a Notice of Utilization, which is the official Medicare determination. If you still disagree, you can appeal by following the instructions on the notice.

Appeals concerning nonhospital services covered under Medicare hospital insurance (including a few inpatient hospital matters not handled by PROs) are handled by the private insurance companies, called intermediaries. If you disagree with an intermediary's initial decision, you have 60 days to request a reconsideration. You can write directly to the intermediary or submit your request through the Social Security Administration. Then, if you disagree with the reconsideration and the amount in question is $100 or more, you have 60 days to request a hearing by an administrative law judge. Cases involving $1,000 or more can be appealed to a federal court.

Note: To meet the $100 requirement, you can combine claims that have been reconsidered. Also, two or more people may combine reconsidered claims if their combined claims were denied for the same reason.

Your Right of Refusal

Q. Can I refuse some medical services?

A. Accepting Medicare funds does not require you to accept all treatment. Nor does it mean you are entitled only to limited services simply because you are receiving coverage under Medicare. You have a right to refuse or accept certain medical services, particularly certain extraordinary life-support measures. You must be given written information about your right to make decisions about your medical care if you:

- Are admitted to a Medicare hospital or skilled nursing facility.
- Begin to receive Medicare home health care.
- Enroll in a Medicare-certified hospice or HMO.

Generally, you will be told about your right to accept or refuse medical or surgical treatment. If not, you should discuss this with the health care facility. You will also be informed of your right to make an advance directive containing written instructions that state your choices for health care. In addition, you have the right to name someone to make those choices for you if you become incapacitated. This directive may be called a living will or a durable medical power of attorney. If you have one, you can decline in advance certain treatment that you do not wish to receive. Your treatment choices, however, vary slightly from state to state. A pamphlet titled *Medicare and Advance Directives* is available from the Federal Consumer Information Center, Department WWW, Pueblo, CO 81009; phone (888) 878-3256; Web site: ***www.pueblo.gsa.gov***.

Other Rules That Help Protect You

Skilled nursing facilities

Skilled nursing facilities cannot require you to pay a deposit or other payment as a condition of admission to the facility—unless it is clear that services are not covered by Medicare. (Many still request deposits in the amount of the Day 20 through Day 100 co-payment.) If you are already a patient in a skilled nursing facility and the staff at the facility decides that you no longer need the level of skilled care covered by Medicare, they must notify you immediately.

If you disagree with this decision, the facility must submit your claim at your request to Medicare for an official decision on coverage. The facility may not require you to pay a deposit until Medicare issues its decision. You must pay for any co-insurance while your claim is being processed and for services that are never covered by Medicare. Also, if you disagree with a decision on the amount Medicare will pay on a claim or whether services you receive are covered, you always have the right to appeal.

If you want to file a complaint about a skilled nursing facility's treatment of patients or other conditions, contact the state survey agency. While you are at the facility, you can look at a copy of the survey agency's latest certification report.

Medicare Summary Notice

After your doctor, provider or supplier sends in a Part B claim, Medicare will send you a Medicare Summary Notice, which tells you its decision on the claim. The notice shows what the charges were, what Medicare approved, your co-payment, the amount Medicare is paying, and whether your $100 annual deductible has not been met. If the doctor, provider or supplier does not take assignment, the notice will show what the limiting charge is. The summary notice also gives the address and phone number for contacting the Medicare carrier.

You should read your notices carefully. If you believe that payments were made for services or supplies you didn't receive, or that payments are questionable for some other reason, call or write to your carrier. Many carriers have installed an automated answering system to help make their responses faster and more accurate.

Note: If a Medicare claim is disallowed, you may be entitled to a waiver of liability in the (unlikely) event that you did not know the services were excluded from coverage.

Your rights under the Privacy Act

Under the Privacy Act, all federal agencies must safeguard information they collect about the people they serve. When CMS asks you to fill out forms giving information about yourself to Medicare, CMS must:

- Explain why it is collecting the information.
- Tell you to whom it plans to give the information.
- Tell you whether you must, by law, give the information.

When you give Medicare information, you are allowed to review your records for accuracy and make corrections if you believe there are errors. The Privacy Act also allows the government to verify the information you give to CMS by using computer matches with other federal or state agencies. If CMS does computer matches, it must tell you it has done so and give you a chance to protest the findings. Information about such matches will be on all the forms you fill out.

Note: Medicare carriers and intermediaries must follow Privacy Act rules. Except under limited circumstances, Medicare contractors may not discuss personal information about you with your family members or others who write or telephone on your behalf unless you give the contractors written permission.

When Protection Ends . . .

For people age 65 and older

If you have Part A hospital insurance based on your spouse's work record, your protection will end if you get a divorce during the first 10 years of marriage. But if you have Part A based on your own work record, your protection will continue as long as you live. If you are buying Part A insurance by paying monthly premiums, you will lose it if you cancel your Part B insurance. Those who buy Part A must also enroll and pay the premium for Part B; however, they can cancel Part A and still continue to buy Part B.

Your Part B protection will stop if your premiums are not paid (normally you will have a 90-day grace period in which to pay your overdue premiums) or if you voluntarily cancel. If you are thinking about canceling Part B, remember that you may not be able to get private insurance that offers the same protection.

For people with disabilities

If you have Medicare because you are disabled, your protection will end if you recover from your disability before age 65.

What if you are disabled and return to work? Under a law passed at the end of 1999, you will be allowed to continue your premium-free Part A coverage for eight and a half years. The Work Incentives Improvement Act extends Part A hospital coverage for an additional four and a half years beyond the 48 months provided under prior law for Social Security disability beneficiaries. Your Part B coverage will also continue as long as you keep paying the monthly premiums.

The law also provides grants that encourage states to allow disabled workers to buy into Medicaid, the state-federal health program for the poor, by paying sliding-scale premiums based on their income.

For people with permanent kidney failure

If you have Medicare because of permanent kidney failure, your protection will end 12 months after the month when maintenance dialysis treatment stops or 36 months after the month you have a kidney transplant. Your Medicare Part B protection could stop before that if you fail to pay the premiums or if you decide to cancel the coverage.

'An Important Message From Medicare'

Your Rights As a Medicare Hospital Patient

You have the right to receive all the hospital care that is necessary for the proper diagnosis and treatment of your illness or injury. According to federal law, **your discharge date must be determined solely by your medical needs,** not by DRGs (Diagnostic Related Group payments) or Medicare payments.

You have the right to be fully informed about decisions affecting your Medicare coverage and payment for your hospital stay and for any posthospital services.

You have the right to request a review by a Peer Review Organization of any written Notice of Noncoverage that you receive from the hospital stating that Medicare will no longer pay for your hospital care. Peer Review Organizations (PROs) are groups of doctors who are paid by the federal government to review medical necessity, appropriateness and quality of hospital treatment furnished to Medicare patients. The phone number and address of the PRO for your area are:

____

[This will be filled in by the hospital.]

Talk to Your Doctor About Your Stay in the Hospital

You and your doctor know more about your condition and your health needs than anyone else. Decisions about your medical treatment should be made between you and your doctor. If you have any questions about your medical treatment, your need for continued hospital care, your discharge or your need for possible posthospital care, **don't hesitate to ask your doctor.** The hospital's patient representative or social worker will also help you with your questions and concerns about hospital services.

If You Think You Are Being Asked to Leave the Hospital Too Soon

Ask a hospital representative for a written notice of explanation immediately, if you have not already received one. This notice is called a Notice of Noncoverage. You must have this Notice of Noncoverage if you wish to exercise your right to request a review by the PRO. The Notice of Noncoverage will state that either your doctor or the PRO agrees with the hospital's decision that Medicare will no longer pay for your hospital care.

If the hospital and your doctor agree, the PRO does not review your case before a Notice of Noncoverage is issued. But the PRO will respond to your request for a review of your Notice of Noncoverage and seek your opinion. You cannot be made to pay for your hospital care until the PRO makes its decision, if you request the review by noon of the first workday after you receive the Notice of Noncoverage.

If the hospital and your doctor disagree, the hospital may request the PRO to review your case. If it does make such a request, the hospital is required to send you a notice to that effect. In this situation, the PRO must agree with the hospital or the hospital cannot issue a Notice of Noncoverage. You may request that the PRO reconsider your case after you receive a Notice of Noncoverage, but since the PRO has already reviewed your case once, you may have to pay for at least one day of hospital care before the PRO completes this reconsideration.

If you do not request a review, the hospital may bill you for all the costs of your stay, beginning with the third day after you receive the Notice of Noncoverage. The hospital, however, cannot charge you for care unless it provides you with a Notice of Noncoverage.

How to Request a Review of the Notice of Noncoverage

If the Notice of Noncoverage states that your physician agrees with the hospital's decision: You must make your request for review to the PRO by **noon of the first workday** after you receive the Notice of Noncoverage by contacting the PRO by phone or in writing. The PRO must ask for your views about your case before making its decision. The PRO will inform you by phone and in writing of its decision on the review.

If the PRO agrees with the Notice of Noncoverage, you may be billed for all costs of your stay, beginning at noon of the day after you receive the PRO's decision. Thus, you will not be responsible for the cost of hospital care before you receive the PRO's decision.

If the Notice of Noncoverage states that the PRO agrees with the hospital's decision: You should make your request for reconsideration to the PRO immediately upon receipt of the Notice of Noncoverage by contacting the PRO by phone or in writing. The PRO can take up to three working days from receipt of your request to complete the review. The PRO will inform you in writing of its decision on the review.

Since the PRO has already reviewed your case once, prior to the issuance of the Notice of Noncoverage, the hospital is permitted to begin billing you for the cost of your stay beginning with the third calendar day after you receive your Notice of Noncoverage, **even if the PRO has not completed its review.**

Thus, if the PRO continues to agree with the Notice of Noncoverage, you may have to pay for at least one day of hospital care.

Note: The process described above is called "immediate review." If you miss the deadline for this immediate review while you are in the hospital, you may still request a review of Medicare's decision no longer to pay for your care at any point during your hospital stay or after you have left the hospital. The Notice of Noncoverage will tell you how to request this review.

Posthospital Care

When your doctor determines that you no longer need all the specialized services provided in a hospital, but you still require medical care, he or she may discharge you to a skilled nursing facility or home care. The discharge planner at the hospital will help arrange for the services you may need after your discharge. Medicare and supplemental insurance policies have limited coverage for skilled nursing facility care and home health care. Therefore, you should find out which services will or will not be covered and how payment will be made. Consult with your doctor, hospital discharge planner, patient representative and your family in making preparations for care after you leave the hospital. Don't hesitate to ask questions.

Acknowledgment of Receipt: My signature merely acknowledges my receipt of this message from *[name of hospital]* on *[date]* and does not waive any of my rights to request a review or make me liable for any payment.

____

[Signature of beneficiary or person acting on behalf of beneficiary]

____

[Date of receipt]

Appendix I: Further Information

Additional publications about health care coverage and long-term care are available to older Americans and their adult children from a variety of government agencies and organizations, including the following:

AARP
601 E St. NW
Washington, DC 20049
(800) 424-3410
www.aarp.org

American Association of Homes and Services for the Aging
901 E St. NW, Suite 500
Washington, DC 20004-2011
(202) 783-2242
www.aahsa.org

American Health Care Association
1201 L St. NW
Washington, DC 20005
(800) 321-0343
(202) 842-4444
www.ahca.org

Centers for Medicare & Medicaid Services (CMS)
7500 Security Blvd.
Baltimore, MD 21244
Medicare hotline:
(800) 633-4227
www.medicare.gov

Families USA
1334 G St. NW
Washington, DC 20005
(202) 628-3030
www.familiesusa.org

Federal Consumer Information Center
Department WWW
Pueblo, CO 81009
(888) 878-3256
www.pueblo.gsa.gov

National Association of Area Agencies on Aging
927 15th St. NW
6th Floor
Washington, DC 20005
(202) 296-8130
www.n4a.org

National Association of Insurance Commissioners
2301 McGee, Suite 800
Kansas City, MO 64108
(816) 842-3600
www.naic.org

National Consumers League
1701 K St. NW
Suite 1201
Washington, DC 20006
(202) 835-3323
www.natlconsumersleague.org

National Council on the Aging
409 3rd St. SW, Suite 200
Washington, DC 20024
(202) 479-1200
www.ncoa.org

***Related Publications From* National Institute of Business Management:**

Social Security: Your 'Hidden' Benefits and How to Claim Them

Elder Care: Caring for Your Aging Loved Ones

Your Children, Your Heirs

Book of Trusts

Essential Guide for Estate Executors, Guardians and Trustees

Retirement Tax Guide

How to Survive a Catastrophic Illness Without Going Broke

To order, phone (800) 543-2055 or visit *www.nibm.net*

Appendix II: State Insurance Regulators

Each state and territory has its own laws and regulations governing all types of insurance. The offices listed in this section are responsible for enforcing those laws, as well as for providing the public with information about insurance.

The 800 numbers listed below can be used only in the states or service areas indicated. Phone numbers change frequently. Please be sure to verify these numbers with your local directory assistance.

Alabama
Dept. of Insurance
Consumer Service Div.
201 Monroe St.
Suite 1700
Montgomery, AL 36104-3351
(334) 269-3550

Alaska
Div. of Insurance
3601 C St., Suite 1324
Anchorage, AK 99503-5948
(907) 269-7900

Arizona
Dept. of Insurance
2910 N. 44th St., Suite 210
Phoenix, AZ 85018-7256
(602) 912-8444

Arkansas
Dept. of Insurance
1200 W. 3rd St.
Little Rock, AR 72201-1904
(800) 282-5494
(501) 371-2600

California
Dept. of Insurance
Consumer Communications Bureau
300 S. Spring St., South Tower
Los Angeles, CA 90013
(213) 897-8921

Colorado
Div. of Insurance
1560 Broadway
Suite 850
Denver, CO 80202-4942
(303) 894-7499
(800) 930-3745

Connecticut
Dept. of Insurance
Consumer Affairs
P.O. Box 816
153 Market St.
11th Floor
Hartford, CT 06142-0816
(800) 203-3447

Delaware
Dept. of Insurance
Rodney Bldg.
841 Silver Lake Blvd.
Dover, DE 19904
(302) 739-4251

District of Columbia
Dept. of Insurance
810 First St. NE, Suite 701
Washington, DC 20002
(202) 727-8000, ext. 3018

Florida
Office of Insurance Regulation
State Capitol, Plaza Level 11
Tallahassee, FL 32399-0300
(800) 342-2762

Georgia
Dept. of Insurance
2 Martin Luther King Jr. Dr.
Floyd Memorial Bldg.
704 West Tower
Atlanta, GA 30334-9008
(800) 656-2298

Hawaii
Insurance Div.
Dept. of Commerce &
Consumer Affairs
250 S. King St., 5th Floor
Honolulu, HI 96813-4505
(808) 586-2790

Idaho
Dept. of Insurance
700 W. State St., 3rd Floor
Boise, ID 83720-0043
(208) 334-4250
(800) 721-3272

Illinois
Dept. of Insurance
320 W. Washington St.
4th Floor
Springfield, IL 62767-0001
(217) 782-4515
100 W. Randolph St.
Suite 15-100
Chicago, IL 60601-3251
(312) 814-2420

Indiana
Dept. of Insurance
311 W. Washington St.
Suite 300
Indianapolis, IN 46204-2787
(800) 622-4461
(317) 232-2385

Iowa
Div. of Insurance
330 E. Maple St.
Des Moines, IA 50319-0001
(515) 281-5705

Kansas
Insurance Division
420 SW 9th St.
Topeka, KS 66612-1678
(800) 432-2484
(785) 296-7801

Kentucky
Dept. of Insurance
215 W. Main St.
P.O. Box 517
Frankfort, KY 40602-0517
(800) 595-6053

Louisiana
Dept. of Insurance
950 N. 5th St.
Baton Rouge, LA 70804-9214
(800) 259-5301
(225) 343-4834

Maine
Bureau of Insurance
State Office Bldg. Station 34
Augusta, ME 04333-0034
(207) 624-8475

Maryland
Insurance Administration
525 St. Paul Place
Stanbalt Bldg., 7th Floor
Baltimore, MD 21202-2272
(800) 492-6116

Massachusetts
Div. of Insurance
One South Station, 5th Floor
Boston, MA 02110-2223
(617) 521-7794

Michigan
Financial and Insurance
Services
611 W. Ottawa St.
2nd Floor North
Lansing, MI 48933-1020
(517) 373-0220

Minnesota
Insurance Div.
Dept. of Commerce
133 E. 7th St.
Suite 200
St. Paul, MN 55101-2145
(651) 296-2488

Mississippi
Dept. of Insurance
Consumer Assistance Div.
P.O. Box 79
Jackson, MS 39205
(601) 359-3569

Missouri
Dept. of Insurance
301 W. High St., 6 North
Jefferson City, MO 65102-0690
(800) 726-7390
(573) 751-4126

Montana
Dept. of Insurance
840 Helena Ave.
Helena, MT 59601-4009
(800) 332-6148

Nebraska
Dept. of Insurance
941 O St., Suite 400
Lincoln, NE 68508-3690
(402) 471-2201

Nevada
Div. of Insurance
1665 Hot Springs Rd.
Suite 152
Carson City, NV 89706
(800) 992-0900
(775) 687-7690

New Hampshire
Dept. of Insurance
56 Old Suncook Rd.
Concord, NH 03301
(800) 852-3416
(603) 271-2261

New Jersey
Dept. of Insurance
20 W. State St., CN325
Trenton, NJ 08625-0325
(609) 633-7667

New Mexico
Dept. of Insurance
P.O. Box 1269
Santa Fe, NM 87504-1269
(505) 827-4601

New York
Dept. of Insurance
Agency Bldg. 1
Empire State Plaza
Albany, NY 12257-0001
(800) 342-3736
(518) 474-6600
25 Beaver St.
New York, NY 10004-2319
(212) 480-6400

North Carolina
Dept. of Insurance
P.O. Box 26387
Raleigh, NC 27611-6387
(800) 662-7777
(919) 733-7349

North Dakota
Dept. of Insurance
600 E. Boulevard
Bismarck, ND 58505-0320
(800) 247-0560
(701) 328-2440

Ohio
Dept. of Insurance
Consumer Services Div.
2100 Stella Ct.
Columbus, OH 43215-1067
(800) 686-1526
(614) 644-3378

Oklahoma
Dept. of Insurance
3814 N. Santa Fe
Oklahoma City, OK 73118
(800) 522-0071
(405) 521-2828

Oregon
Div. of Insurance
350 Winter St. NE
Salem, OR 97310-3883
(503) 947-7984
(888) 877-4894

Pennsylvania
Dept. of Insurance
Consumer Services Bureau
1321 Strawberry Square
Harrisburg, PA 17120
(877) 881-6388

Rhode Island
Insurance Div.
233 Richmond St., Suite 233
Providence, RI 02903-4233
(401) 222-2223

South Carolina
Dept. of Insurance
1612 Marion St.
P.O. Box 100105
Columbia, SC 29202-3105
(800) 768-3467
(803) 737-6180

South Dakota
Div. of Insurance
118 W. Capitol Ave.
Pierre, SD 57501-2000
(605) 773-3563

Tennessee
Dept. of Commerce &
Insurance
500 James Robertson Pkwy.
Nashville, TN 37243-0565
(800) 525-2816
(615) 741-2241

Texas
Dept. of Insurance
333 Guadalupe St.
P.O. Box 149104
Austin, TX 78714-9104
(800) 252-3439
(512) 463-6169

Utah
Dept. of Insurance
3110 State Office Bldg.
Salt Lake City, UT 84114-1201
(800) 439-3805
(801) 538-3826

Vermont
Dept. of Insurance
89 Main St.
Drawer 20
Montpelier, VT 05620-3101
(800) 964-1784

Virginia
Bureau of Insurance
State Corporation
Commission
P.O. Box 1157
Richmond, VA 23218
(800) 552-7945
(804) 371-9967

Washington
Office of the Insurance
Commissioner
P.O. Box 40255
Olympia, WA 98504-0255
(360) 753-3613
(800) 562-6900

West Virginia
Dept. of Insurance
P.O. Box 50540
Charleston, WV 25305-0540
(800) 642-9004
(304) 558-3354

Wisconsin
Office of Commissioner
of Insurance
121 E. Wilson
Madison, WI 53702
(800) 236-8517
(608) 266-0103

Wyoming
Dept. of Insurance
Herschler Bldg.
122 W. 25th St., 3rd East
Cheyenne, WY 82002-0440
(800) 438-5768
(307) 777-7401

American Samoa
Insurance Commissioner
Office of the Governor
Pago Pago, AS 96799-9999
011 (684) 633-4116

Guam
Dept. of Revenue & Taxation
Building 13-3, 1st Floor
Mariner Ave.
Tiyan, Barrigada, GU 96913
011 (671) 475-1843

Puerto Rico
Department of Insurance
Cobian's Plaza Bldg.
1607 Ponce de Leon Ave.
Santurce, PR 00909
(787) 722-8686

Virgin Islands
Div. of Banking and Insurance
Kongen's Gade #18
St. Thomas, VI 00820
(340) 774-7166

Appendix III: State Agencies on Aging

The offices listed in this section are responsible for coordinating services for the senior citizens in their states or territories.

The 800 numbers listed below can be used only in the states or service areas indicated. Phone numbers change frequently. Please be sure to verify these numbers with your local directory assistance.

Alabama
Alabama Dept.
of Senior Services
RSA Plaza
Suite 470
770 Washington Ave.
Montgomery, AL 36130-1851
(800) 243-5463
(334) 242-5743

Alaska
Alaska Commission
on Aging
Div. of Senior Services
Dept. of Administration
P.O. Box 110209
Juneau, AK 99811-0209
(907) 465-3250

Arizona
Aging & Adult
Administration
Dept. of Economic Security
1789 W. Jefferson St.
Suite 950A
Phoenix, AZ 85007-3202
(602) 542-4446

Arkansas
Aging & Adult Services Div.
Arkansas Dept. of Human
Services
P.O. Box 1437
1417 Donaghey Plaza South
Little Rock, AR 72203-1437
(501) 682-2441

California
Dept. of Aging
1600 K St.
Sacramento, CA 95814-4020
(916) 322-5290

Colorado
Aging and Adult
Services Div.
Dept. of Social Services
110 16th St., Suite 200
Denver, CO 80202
(303) 620-4147

Connecticut
Div. of Elderly Services
25 Sigourney St., 10th Floor
Hartford, CT 06106-5033
(800) 443-9946
(860) 424-5277

Delaware
Div. of Services for
Aging and Adults With
Physical Disabilities
Dept. of Health &
Social Services
1901 N. DuPont Highway
New Castle, DE 19720-1100
(302) 577-4791

District of Columbia
Office on Aging
441 4th St. NW, Suite 900 S.
Washington, DC 20001-2700
(202) 724-5622

Florida
Dept. of Elder Affairs
4040 Esplanade Way, Suite 152
Tallahassee, FL 32399-7000
(904) 414-2000

Georgia
Div. of Aging Services
Dept. of Human Resources
2 Peachtree St. NE
Suite 36-385
Atlanta, GA 30303-3176
(404) 657-5258

Hawaii
Executive Office on Aging
250 S. Hotel St., Suite 109
Honolulu, HI 96813-2831
(808) 586-0100

Idaho
Commission on Aging
P.O. Box 83720
Boise, ID 83720-0007
(208) 334-3833

Illinois
Dept. on Aging
421 E. Capitol Ave.
Suite 100
Springfield, IL 62701-1789
(800) 252-8966
Chicago office:
(312) 814-2630

Indiana
Disability, Aging &
Rehabilitative Services Div.
Family and Social Services
402 W. Washington St.
P.O. Box 7083
Indianapolis, IN 46207-7083
(800) 545-7763
(317) 232-7020

Iowa
Dept. of Elder Affairs
Clemens Bldg., 3rd Floor
200 10th St.
Des Moines, IA 50309-3609
(515) 281-4646

Kansas
Dept. on Aging
503 S. Kansas Ave.
Topeka, KS 66603-3404
(785) 296-4986

Kentucky
Office of Aging Services
Cabinet for Families
and Children
275 E. Main St., 6 West
Frankfort, KY 40621-0001
(502) 564-6930

Louisiana
Governor's Office
of Elderly Affairs
P.O. Box 80374
Baton Rouge, LA 70898-0374
(504) 342-7100

Maine
Bureau of Elder &
Adult Services
Dept. of Human Services
35 Anthony Ave.
State House, Station 11
Augusta, ME 04333-3011
(207) 624-5335

Maryland
Dept. of Aging
State Office Building
Room 1007
301 W. Preston St.
Baltimore, MD 21201-2374
(410) 767-1100

Massachusetts
Executive Office of
Elder Affairs
One Ashburton Place
5th Floor
Boston, MA 02108-1518
(800) 882-2003
(617) 727-7750

Michigan
Office of Services to the Aging
P.O. Box 30676
Lansing, MI 48909
(517) 373-8230

Minnesota
Board on Aging
444 Lafayette Rd.
St. Paul, MN 55155-3843
(800) 882-6262
(651) 296-1531

Mississippi
Aging & Adult Services Div.
750 N. State St.
Jackson, MS 39202-3033
(800) 948-3090
(601) 359-4925

Missouri
Div. on Aging
Dept. of Social Services
P.O. Box 1337
615 Howerton Court
Jefferson City, MO 65102-1337
(573) 751-3082

Montana
Senior and Long-Term
Care Div.
Dept. of Public Health &
Human Services
P.O. Box 4210
111 Sanders, Room 211
Helena, MT 59620
(800) 332-2272
(406) 444-7788

Nebraska
Div. on Aging
P.O. Box 95044
1343 M St.
Lincoln, NE 68509-5044
(402) 471-2307

Nevada
Div. for Aging Services
Dept. of Human Resources
3416 Goni Rd.
Bldg. D
Carson City, NV 89706
(775) 687-4210

New Hampshire
Div. of Health and Human
Services
State Office Park South
129 Pleasant St.
Brown Bldg. 1
Concord, NH 03301-3843
(603) 271-4680

New Jersey
Div. of Senior Affairs
Dept. of Health and Senior
Services
P.O. Box 807
Trenton, NJ 08625-0807
(800) 792-8820
(609) 588-3141

New Mexico
State Agency on Aging
La Villa Rivera Bldg.
228 E. Palace Ave.
Santa Fe, NM 87501-2013
(800) 432-2080
(505) 827-7640

New York
Office for the Aging
2 Empire State Plaza
Albany, NY 12223-1251
(800) 342-9871
(518) 474-5731

North Carolina
Div. of Aging
2101 Mail Service Center
Raleigh, NC 27699-2101
(919) 733-3983

North Dakota
Dept. of Human Services
Aging Services Div.
600 S. 2nd St., Suite 1C
Bismarck, ND 58504-7070
(701) 328-8910
(800) 451-8693

Ohio
Dept. of Aging
50 W. Broad St., 9th Floor
Columbus, OH 43215-5928
(800) 282-1206
(614) 466-5500

Oklahoma
Aging Services Div.
Dept. of Human Services
P.O. Box 25352
312 NE 28th St.
Oklahoma City, OK 73125-0352
(405) 521-2281

Oregon
Senior & Disabled
Services Div.
500 Summer St. NE
Salem, OR 97310-1015
(800) 232-8096
(503) 945-5811

Pennsylvania
Dept. of Aging
555 Walnut St., 5th Floor
Harrisburg, PA 17101-1919
(717) 783-1550

Rhode Island
Dept. of Elderly Affairs
160 Pine St.
Providence, RI 02903-3708
(401) 277-2858

South Carolina
Office of Senior and
Long-Term Care Services
P.O. Box 8206
Columbia, SC 29202-8206
(803) 898-2501

South Dakota
Office of Adult
Services & Aging
700 Governors Dr.
Pierre, SD 57501-2291
(605) 773-3656

Tennessee
Commission on Aging
500 Deaderick St., 9th Floor
Nashville, TN 37243-0860
(615) 741-2056

Texas
Dept. on Aging
4900 N. Lamar, 4th Floor
Austin, TX 78751-2316
(800) 252-9240
(512) 424-6840

Utah
Aging & Adult Services
P.O. Box 45500
120 N. 200 West
Salt Lake City, UT 84145-0500
(801) 534-3910

Vermont
Dept. of Aging &
Disabilities
103 S. Main St.
Waterbury, VT 05671-2301
(802) 241-2400

Virginia
Dept. for the Aging
1600 Forest Ave., Suite 102
Richmond, VA 23229
(800) 552-4464
(804) 662-9333

Washington
Aging & Adult
Services Admin.
Dept. of Social &
Health Services
P.O. Box 45050
Olympia, WA 98504-5050
(360) 493-2500
(800) 422-3263

West Virginia
Bureau of Senior Services
Holly Grove, Bldg. 10
1900 Kanawha Blvd. East
Charleston, WV 25305-0160
(304) 558-3317

Wisconsin
Bureau of Aging
Dept. of Health &
Family Services
P.O. Box 7851
Madison, WI 53707-7851
(800) 242-1060
(608) 266-2536

Wyoming
Dept. of Health
Office on Aging
117 Hathaway Bldg.
Room 139
Cheyenne, WY 82002-0710
(800) 442-2766
(307) 777-7986

American Samoa
Territorial Admin. on Aging
Government of American
Samoa
Pago Pago, AS 96799-9999
011 (684) 633-2207
fax 011 (684) 633-2533

Guam
Div. of Senior Citizens
Dept. of Public Health &
Social Services
P.O. Box 2816
Agana, GU 96910
011 (671) 475-0263
fax 011 (671) 477-2930

Marshall Islands
State Agency on Aging
Dept. of Social Services
Republic of the
Marshall Islands
Marjuro, Marshall Islands
96960-9999

Micronesia
State Agency on Aging
Office of Health Services
Federated States of
Micronesia
Ponape, E.C.I. 96941

Northern Mariana Islands
CNMI Office on Aging
P.O. Box 2178
Commonwealth of the
Northern Mariana Islands
Saipan, MP 96950-9999
011 (670) 233-1320
fax 011 (670) 233-1327

Palau
State Agency on Aging
Republic of Palau
Koror, PW 96940-9999
011 (680) 488-2736
fax 011 (680) 488-1662

Puerto Rico
Governor's Office of
Elderly Affairs
P.O. Box 50063
San Juan, PR 00902-6263
(787) 721-5710
fax (787) 721-6510

Virgin Islands
Dept. of Human Services
Knud Hansen Complex
Bldg. A
1303 Hospital Ground
Charlotte Amalie, VI
00802-6722
(340) 774-0930
fax (340) 774-3466

National Institute of Business Management

TOP-SELLING SPECIAL REPORTS

	Special Report Title	Price	Code	Qty.	Total Cost
	Business Management				
	Cashing Out: How to Sell Your Business for Top Dollar	$39.95	N269	____	______
	Best Practices: Elder Care	$29.95	N336	____	______
READER FAVORITE	*Taming the Paper Monster: Records Management, Compliance and File Security*	$39.95	N247	____	______
	Keeping Customers for Life	$39.95	N254	____	______
	Super Sales Strategies	$34.95	N259	____	______
	Building a Super Sales Team	$34.95	N260	____	______
	Super Sales Strategies and *Building a Super Sales Team*—***Special Combo Price***	$59.95	N263	____	______
	Business Succession Planning	$49.95	N288	____	______
	Business Is War: 9 Classic Rules of War for Winning Big in Business	$29.95	N282	____	______
	Family Business Survival Kit: Preserve Your Legacy for Generations	$39.95	N335	____	______
	Financial Planning & Tax Reduction				
	Essential Guide for Estate Executors, Guardians and Trustees	$39.95	N085	____	______
	How to Build & Tax-Proof Your Estate	$39.95	N089	____	______
	How to Survive a Catastrophic Illness Without Going Broke	$49.95	N087	____	______
READER FAVORITE	*The Book of Trusts*	$49.95	N186	____	______
	Stealth Tax Strategies for Business Owners and Managers	$39.95	N226	____	______
	175 Tax Reduction Strategies	$59.95	N181	____	______
	Anti-Audit Warfare	$39.95	N180	____	______
	Surprise Tax Windfall	$29.95	N285	____	______
	Tax-Wise Investment Strategies	$29.95	N293	____	______
	Management Skills				
READER FAVORITE	*Mastering Business Finance*	$39.95	N022	____	______
	Mastering Business Etiquette & Protocol	$29.95	N107	____	______
	Mastering Office Politics	$29.95	N028	____	______
	Mastering Business Presentations	$39.95	N338	____	______
	Mastering Business Negotiation	$39.95	N281	____	______
READER FAVORITE	*Difficult People at Work*	$29.95	N115	____	______
	Manager's Guide to Effective, Legal Performance Reviews	$39.95	N246	____	______
	The Art of Selling Your Ideas	$39.95	N070	____	______
	The Manager's Answer Book	$29.95	N340	____	______
	How to Get Twice As Much Done in Half As Much Time	$29.95	N114	____	______
	The Ultimate Cost-Cutting Guide for Small Business	$24.95	N296	____	______
	The Black Book of Executive Politics, by Z	$39.95	N284	____	______
	Human Resources				
	The Book of Company Policies	$59.95	N278	____	______
	Bullet-Proof Your Employee Handbook	$29.95	N279	____	______
	Employer's Practical Legal Guide: (revised annually) Plain Language About Current Employment Law	$137.00	N283	____	______
	Complete Guide to Employee Benefits	$79.95	N301	____	______
	444 Slam-Dunk Recruiting Strategies	$39.95	N308	____	______

Please continue to the next page for more Special Report titles...

NATIONAL INSTITUTE OF BUSINESS MANAGEMENT

SPECIAL REPORT TITLE	PRICE	CODE	QTY.	TOTAL COST
Do-It-Yourself Employee Manual	$279.00	N077	____	______
Small Business Legal Series:				
You and the ADA	$29.95	N264	____	______
Sexual Harassment	$29.95	N265	____	______
Using Independent Contractors	$29.95	N268	____	______
You and the FMLA	$29.95	N266	____	______
You and the FLSA	$29.95	N309	____	______
Special Combo Price for All 5 Reports	$103.95	N334	____	______
READER FAVORITE *Fire at Will*	$29.95	N235	____	______
Hire at Will	$19.95	N236	____	______
Fire at Will and *Hire at Will*—***Special Combo Price***	$44.90	N237	____	______
Great Hires—Every Time	$39.95	N258	____	______
The Flexible Work Force	$39.95	N221	____	______
Wanted: A Few Good Employee Incentives	$39.95	N255	____	______
440 Ways to Get More Out of Your Employees	$29.95	N016	____	______
RETIREMENT PLANNING				
READER FAVORITE *Social Security: Your "Hidden" Benefits and How to Claim Them (revised annually)*	$49.95	N188	____	______
The Medicare Guide (revised annually)	$39.95	N189	____	______
Social Security and *Medicare Guide*—***Special Combo Price***	$79.95	N187	____	______
Retirement Tax Guide	$39.95	N209	____	______
Your Children, Your Heirs: An Estate Planning Guide	$39.95	N053	____	______
Elder Care: Caring for Your Aging Loved Ones	$39.95	N214	____	______

- -

Please call for information on other topics.

To order, simply fill in the number of copies you want for each report and mail in this form.

100% Money-Back Guarantee

Payment options:

☐ Check enclosed (payable to: NIBM)

☐ Please charge my credit card: ☐ Visa ☐ MasterCard ☐ AmEx ☐ Discover

Card #________________________ Exp. Date ____________

Signature________________________________

Name________________________ (please print)

Title ________________________________

Firm ________________________________

Address ________________________________

City____________________ State ________ ZIP____________

Daytime Phone (______) ____________ Fax (______)____________

Please mail to: National Institute of Business Management, P.O. Box 9070, McLean, VA 22102-0070.

Please allow 3 weeks for delivery.

ORDER TOTAL ____ $________

$4.50 S&H (1st copy)
*$5.50 S&H (for special combo) $________

S&H add'l copies ($1.50 each) $________

VA residents add 4.5% sales tax $________

Canada: please add GST/HST (if applicable) $________

TOTAL $________

Payable in U.S. dollars or Canadian equivalent.

Ask for Special Offer S00420.

For faster delivery of your order:

call
(800) 543-2055

fax
(703) 905-8040

or go to
www.nibm.net

Rev. 10/02